Ruby MacDonald's Forty-Plus and Feeling Fabulous Book

Ruby MacDonald's Forty-Plus and Feeling Fabulous Book

Ruby MacDonald

Fleming H. Revell Company
Old Tappan, New Jersey

Library of Congress Cataloging in Publication Data
MacDonald, Ruby.
Ruby MacDonald's Forty-plus and feeling
fabulous book.
1. Middle aged women—Conduct of life.
I. Title.
BJ1610.M28   158'.1'024042   82-3844
ISBN 0-8007-1308-7   AACR2

TO Tim and Tobi,
 who helped create my ageless attitude.
TO Shannon, Debbie, and Mike,
 who continue to stimulate my ageless attitude.
TO Tom,
 the fabulous husband God sent to me at mid-life, who has taught me so much about love and life. Without his undying support and encouragement, this book would still be only a thought.

Contents

Part V Surviving a Divorce

Part VI Getting the Most out of This Book

Acknowledgments

My special thanks:

TO Fritz Ridenour, my patient, encouraging editor, who spent countless hours trying to keep his ageless attitude while he organized all the nuts and bolts, so we could create a fabulous book at forty-plus.

TO the warm, congenial people at Fleming H. Revell, who were a joy to work with.

TO Lauraine Snelling and Pat Rushford, my gently ruthless, but loving, critique group.

TO the Portland support group: Susan Fletcher, Linda Freedman, and Rae Ludwig.

TO Shirley Lawson, L.P.N.; Bev Roberts, R.N.; Otis F. Burris, M.D.; and Ben H. McGough, Jr., M.D.; for taking time from their busy schedules to help me with medical research.

TO my many friends and acquaintances who willingly shared their lives and filled me with new energy through their interest and enthusiasm.

TO Christiane McLachlan at Omega Printing, who made this country girl feel like a celebrity as each chapter became a reality.

TO those who shared their talents:
Sydney Craft Rozen, Bob Moser, Yvonne Horn, Lee Roddy.

A very special thanks:

TO the Harry Samuelson family of Ontario, California, who planted the seeds of Christianity in my impressionable young mind so many years ago.

Introduction

Every woman approaching forty, or who is in the forty-plus years, should read this book. I read each chapter with growing interest and enthusiasm, because I feel that Ruby MacDonald's experience and wise counsel can benefit any woman in this general age category.

I have known Ruby for quite a number of years and have seen her grow from an insecure young woman into a poised, confident, self-assured person of fifty. Had I not known better, I would have thought her to be in her thirties when I saw her recently. She has achieved this by applying the principles she sets forth so lucidly in these pages.

Any woman who reads and practices the principles outlined in this book can emulate Ruby's example and make those after-forty years the best years of her life, "the last of life for which the first was made," as Browning put it.

CECIL G. OSBORNE, PH.D., D.D.

Preface

Are you a prisoner of your age?

Everywhere I go, I hear women make reference to their age as a measure of their ability to do or not do something. "I'm too old to ride a bike," my neighbor tells me. "Men don't like women my age—I'm too old," says my attractive divorced friend.

This kind of talk does more than irritate me. At times I get indignant. That's why I've constructed this handbook for all of you who are forty-plus—married, divorced, or single—and want to feel fabulous again. I don't just mean beauty and health tips. We'll talk about those areas too, because they are an important part of feeling fabulous—but the major theme of this book is different. I want you to develop or strengthen what I call an *ageless attitude*. I believe you can become an ageless woman through your thoughts, feelings, and beliefs. As you think, you are. You are as old or as young as you want to think.

You no longer need to think of yourself as old and worn out—you can be *Forty-Plus and Feeling Fabulous* simply by changing your old thought patterns to an ageless attitude.

I haven't always had an ageless attitude. When I was twenty-five, Dr. Norman Vincent Peale made a gigantic impact on my life through his book *The Power of Positive Thinking*. That book changed my life and prepared me for the future, which included meeting and working with Dr. Cecil G. Osborne, director and founder of Westcoast Yokefellows and Burlingame Counseling Center, Burlingame, California.

Through my long involvement in Yokefellows, I owe much
of my ageless attitude to my good friend and teacher, Dr. "O,"
as he is affectionately known.

When I first met Dr. "O," Westcoast Yokefellows was in its
infancy. The church I had visited only once announced its intent to form a pilot group. Because of the void in my life, I
signed up eagerly.

Ten people promised to meet once a week for thirteen
weeks. Slowly, we learned to trust and love one another. As we
did so, we cautiously revealed some of our innermost thoughts
and struggles. As we prayed for one another during the week,
God was the bond of cohesiveness for our group.

I found the small Yokefellows group tremendously exciting
as I grew. I saw that just about everyone struggled with one
kind of problem or another. Since we have learned to wear our
"masks" so well, most people appear to have their lives completely under control. Not so!

Through my participation, study, and attendance at workshops and seminars, I prepared to become a leader of Yokefellow groups. For over ten years, at Covina Methodist Church, I
led and participated in groups for women as well as couples. I
also developed the first Southern California Yokefellow office.

Later, after moving to Washington, I laid the groundwork
for Pacific Northwest Yokefellows and held the first confer-
ence at Warm Beach.

It was through Yokefellows I learned that the message of the
Bible can be a great help in building a positive attitude. Anyone can use the Bible with great benefit, particularly women
who are forty-plus, because the Bible gives principles that
build a strong, abundant life. These principles are a large part
of the Yokefellow discipline and have made me an ageless
woman who is feeling fabulous at a time when many women
feel life is over.

As we progress through this book together, I hope you'll
read it through once to get the idea and generate enthusiasm
for a new way of life. Then I'd like you to go back and read one

chapter at a time. Stay with one chapter until you have learned to make the proposed changes in it a daily part of your life.

Then, as you move on to the next chapter, weave in the ideas from the previous chapters. This is a very special book. It's yours. To get the most out of it, take a yellow felt marker, a red pen, and a pencil. Mark the words and passages that jump out at you. Write in the margins. Make notes in the spaces provided throughout the book. It will be easier to make changes in your life if you capture your thoughts as you go. Thoughts have a way of hiding from you, particularly when they reflect human needs and changes. When you get to the end of this book, you should be well on your way to developing an ageless attitude, being Forty-Plus and Feeling Fabulous.

You'll discover you no longer have to be a prisoner of your age. The years you've lived do not have to dictate your thinking or life-style. It's a truth I've discovered slowly. Today, at age fifty, I'm even more convinced of it.

I feel so strongly about the importance of an ageless attitude that I've been wrongly accused of being an ageist. *Ageist* is a new word in our society. You know what a racist and a sexist are—well, an ageist is one who believes that people become inferior when they have lived a specific number of years.

My friends tell me there is a fine line between my beliefs and those of an ageist. I definitely am not an ageist. But I do hate seeing the way many aging women think, live, and waste away. I'm certainly not against the aged, but *I am* against anyone aging in a negative life-style—having a negative attitude about life—because society says anyone over the age of forty just doesn't have "it" any longer.

We do have "it"—and we can gather more of "it" as the days and years accumulate. We're not only getting older, we're definitely getting better, wiser, and more productive. We have more to contribute to society all through our *growing years.*

I hope your interest in your own life is strong enough to want to explore each chapter with me so you, too, can emerge: FORTY-PLUS AND FEELING FABULOUS.

HOW OLD WUDJA BE IF YA DIDN'T KNOW HOW

O
L
D
Y
A
W
U
Z?

Tricky—fun to read?
It's much more than that.
You can forget it—
Never think about it again
                or
You can write it on your bathroom mirror.
Look at it every day.
Think about it.
Play around with it.
Find yourself some answers.
To one of the most provocative questions you've
    ever been asked.
That's what this book is all about.

How to be more:

A	G	E	L	E	S	S
c	r	n	o	s	e	p
t	a	e	v	s	r	i
i	c	r	a	e	e	r
v	i	g	b	n	n	i
e	o	i	l	t	e	t
	u	z	e	i		u
	s	e		a		a
		d		l		l

than you think you oughta be

17

Part I

Developing the Ageless Attitude

The greatest discovery of my generation is that human beings can alter their lives by altering their attitude of mind.

WILLIAM JAMES

1

The Inner You

You are the light of the world. . . .
let your light . . . *shine. . . .*[1]

I sat talking to my friend Bernice, who had just passed her fortieth birthday. She was confused by the solemn celebration her colleagues had given her. Parties are supposed to be fun. This one left a dark cloud of gloom.

Bernice had been sitting at her desk. The receptionist buzzed her to come out for a moment to tend to an urgent matter. While Bernice was out, someone slipped in. Five huge black balloons floated over her desk when she returned. "Happy Fortieth Birthday!"

Black Friday!

At lunch Bernice's business associates offered their condolences. Bernice wondered if this was the end of the line. It was just another day—not any different from yesterday when she was thirty-nine. But today, all the black thoughts about being forty started taking their toll. Suddenly Bernice felt old. Yesterday she wasn't even aware of her age.

When Bernice finished telling me her story, I congratulated her on being a lively forty and said: "You're just beginning to live."

"I hope so. I was beginning to wonder," she replied. "You're the only one who has congratulated me on having a fortieth birthday—people think of it as a curse."

Too many women believe being forty is a curse instead of a blessing. But being forty-plus is a blessing: because you're still alive—and because you have a choice about how you'll continue to live. Those birthday balloons should have been cheerful yellow, not gloomy black! And I would have attached this poem of mine to warn Bernice about the signs of growing old:

WHAT IS GROWING OLD?

When all you can do is remember
  "the good old days . . ."
When you quit putting your all into whatever
  you're doing . . .
When you think you've learned all there is
  to know . . .
When you stop asking questions . . .
When you no longer wonder how things work . . .
When you're no longer awestruck by a brilliant
  crimson sunset on the water . . .
And the multitude of bright sparkling stars
  in the black velvety night . . .
When you lose the joy of living and can't delight in:
  Seeing the first giant yellow daffodils
    of spring . . .
  Holding a soft, freshly bathed baby
    in your arms and having the scent
    of powder tickle your nose . . .
  Feeling the warmth of a baby's tiny fingers
    as they gently grip one of yours . . .
  Watching the frolics of a cuddly round puppy . . .
When you can no longer laugh at your own mistakes,
And life becomes too serious . . .
That's your clue
YOU ARE GROWING OLD!

Bernice's fortieth birthday signifies she is getting older. But whether or not she wants to grow old in attitude and perspective is *definitely up to her*. If she allows her life to become so serious she can no longer laugh at her own mistakes, that will indeed be the time for those gloomy black balloons.

How to Create an Ageless Attitude

An attitude of feeling old is negative excess baggage at any time of life, not just at forty-plus. My goal in this book is to help you develop or strengthen what I call an *ageless attitude.* An ageless attitude can keep you vital and feeling fabulous. I know you can have an ageless attitude, because I do. And I'm not any different from you. So, let's go for it!

"Okay, Ruby! But where did you get your ageless attitude?" you may be asking.

Well, I'll tell you. For one thing, I believe to be ageless is a gift—a gift from God. But like everything else worthwhile in this life, there's a lot of hard work and persistence involved. Once I realized a new attitude was possible, I had to find ways to change my thinking.

I had help from many people along the way, and I want to share what I have learned. As you become more excited about your ageless attitude, your enthusiasm will become contagious as people notice the change in you and you spread the good word.

Then you'll agree with Joe E. Lewis when he said: "You're only young once—and if you work it right—once is enough."

Once *is* enough! Yes, it's enough because the vitality of youth can be yours no matter what your numerical age. There's no stop sign to halt your growth. Nothing turns you "old" as you round the corner. *Old is in your head!* Old is your state of mind.

In his book *It Takes a Long Time to Become Young,* Garson Kanin quotes that ageless pitcher—a man who held on in the big leagues until the very end of his career—that baseball great—Leroy "Satchel" Paige. Satch asks one of the most provocative questions of all time: "How old would you be if you didn't know how old you was?"

Whenever I ask people that question, smiles spread across their faces. Some laugh; but others ponder the meaning of a question they've never before dared to ask themselves. One woman keeps a typed copy of that question by her kitchen sink as a constant reminder that age is unimportant.

Right now, I'd like you to dwell on Satchel Paige's provocative question. Take as long as necessary. Then jot down the answers that come to mind.

How old would you be if you didn't know how old you are?

Why?

Of course, I have no idea what you thought or wrote. That question affects people differently. Some people write negative things. Some say they would like to be much younger—kids again. One woman of fifty-two wrote "40" and sighed. But the answers tend to show that we have allowed our thinking to trap us inside our chronological age without realizing it. I've found that a change of attitude releases me from any power my age has over me.

Would you like to enter into a world that will free you from being a hostage of your chronological age?

And too, have you ever wondered why some women feel vital and alive at forty-plus while others look as if they've been caught in the worst winter storm of the century?

It's attitude that makes the difference. An ageless attitude can free you to live and enjoy each year of your life with vitality and limitless boundaries.

As I mentioned in the introduction, we live in an ageist society where this ageless attitude does *not* abound. Maggie Kuhn, founder of the Gray Panthers, an organization to help combat prejudice toward aging, has said: "Ageism is the notion that people become inferior because they have lived a specific number of years."[2]

Since that prejudice does exist, instead of seeing yourself as forty and over the hill, I'd rather have *you* see yourself as an ageless woman. You do have that option if you're willing to make some changes.

And it's worth making those changes, because there's something very special about an ageless woman. She's visible in any crowd, but outer beauty and expensive clothing are not a must. Neither are strands of gold around her neck. Her hair may not be in the latest style, but she has "it." And you know, the minute you spot her.

The ageless woman can be forty, fifty, sixty, and beyond. Her chronological age makes no difference. She is the envy of many who know her. Women admire her. Men are drawn to her. Her positive attitude about herself and the vitality of life—how she sees herself in relation to it and the world—are all reflected in her total being: the way she walks, the way she looks, the way she does things, her relationships with other people, and her unmistakable enthusiasm about life.

The ageless woman has discovered that her very own power of mind gives her that elusive fountain of youth for which every woman yearns. And it's free!

Oh, an ageless attitude is not going to restore firm skin, remove wrinkles or gray hair. But those inevitable physical changes won't be enough to stop her from being a confident, ageless woman of today!

I have found that by allowing this positive creative energy to direct my life, the focus on this powerful asset leads to an ageless life-style. This ageless attitude can prevail for an entire lifetime. It's this positive vitality that will let *you* stand out in a crowd and feel fabulous at forty-plus.

Even though women of forty-plus accept their fate of growing older, it's not without inner conflict. Let's face it. No one *enjoys* growing older. It's a difficult adjustment.

Where Does an Ageless Attitude Come From?

Maybe you're wondering how I happened to be lucky enough to discover this eternal fountain of youth. Sometimes desperation leads to restoration.

Let me go back to my high-school days. I turned a very immature seventeen a few weeks after graduation. I suddenly found myself grown-up and bewildered. I didn't know what being grown-up meant. I felt like a stranger in a new land, yet I had to live in that land without knowing how. (That's where many women find themselves in mid-life, too.)

Since my old-fashioned Italian father didn't believe girls needed a college education, I went to work. I tickled the typewriter keys as a typist till I became a secretary. At twenty I married a man my parents urged me not to. The difference in our backgrounds produced nineteen years of intermittent frustration and unhappiness.

At twenty-four I began to see more than a glimpse of the miserable attitudes comprising this five-feet-two-inch frame everyone called Ruby. I needed inner resources desperately, but I was empty. That was the beginning of my long struggle.

In the eighth month of pregnancy I quit my secretarial job to prepare for a new life as mother. A few weeks later Timothy Scott was born—a healthy, blue-eyed, eight-pound baby boy. A month later, I lapsed into postnatal depression.

If you've ever felt lost and helpless, you'll know how I felt. I was scared. I couldn't eat. I couldn't cope well—and I had a precious baby to care for.

In desperation I turned to the doctor who had delivered my little son. I'll never forget that sensitive man. Seeing my devastation, the doctor asked me one simple, but thought-provoking, question: *Do you know that thinking is nothing more than a habit? You can change the way you think if you want to.*

It was as though he handed me a gold bar—heavy and precious. Even though it was twenty-six years ago, I still hear the question that changed me and can change you. That doctor's concern made an impact on my life, the depth of which he can never realize.

Then, seeing that I was totally stunned by the problem, my doctor suggested I read *The Power of Positive Thinking* by Dr. Norman Vincent Peale.

My mind was blotter dry. As I devoured Dr. Peale's book, I absorbed many of the new (to me) constructive ways to think. I began to change, slowly. Daily, I followed that book, page by page. I learned to empty my mind of one negative thought after another. I replaced worry and self-hate with happier, life-building attitudes. *The Power of Positive Thinking* became my guidebook for the next few years. I strongly recommend it, or any of Dr. Peale's many books, as a starting or strengthening point for you.

I had no idea how this new philosophy would stimulate my life. But it established the foundation for my active involvement in Yokefellows and for developing my ageless attitude. Two years later I became a vital Christian with the help of two more people: the Reverend Vickrey Dougherty, then pastor of Covina Methodist Church in Covina, California; and Dr. Cecil Osborne, then minister of Burlingame Baptist Church and counselor, director-founder of Westcoast Yokefellows in Burlingame, California.

As I learned to control my mind and lead it in the direction I wanted my life to go, I developed an ageless attitude filled with positive thoughts about myself, other people, and life. I also developed strength. Much of that strength came through strict discipline of my mind and body. I also learned to understand myself, to make change possible.

A good starting place for self-understanding is a popular-psychology book that makes personality function easier to understand. In his book *I'm OK—You're OK,* Dr. Thomas A. Harris divides personality into three parts—*parent, adult, child*—as shown on the diagram on page 28, which is based on his ideas.

The following is a very brief sketch to help you understand the conflicts you may be experiencing at mid-life. I'll be using Dr. Harris's terminology as we go through it.

It's the *little girl (child)* in you that may be causing some of the disruptions in your life. Since your emotional responses come from your *child,* she will protest when her needs are not

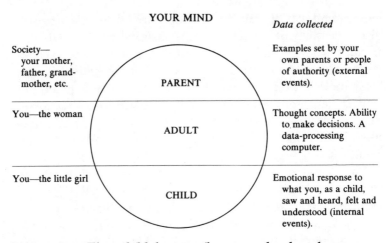

being met. The *child* knows (because she has been programmed by your old attitudes and those of society) that if you get old, she won't be getting the same kind of attention she's been used to, particularly if you are an attractive woman.

Less attention means there won't be as much emotional satisfaction to fill the *child's* needs. (Sometimes the elderly revert back to childish ways, simply to get the attention they once had.) If the *little girl* doesn't get positive strokes, she'll find ways that may be negative to bring attention to herself. That's one reason why early detection of negative attitudes is essential.

Right now, your *child* may feel unloved, unlovely, and unlovable. Those feelings are powerful and may cause you much irritation and frustration.

Your *parent* causes as much trouble if you allow her to. "Let yourself grow old—you can't do anything about it anyway," the *parent* growls at you. Your *parent* is the authority who tries to make you feel guilty if you don't think and do things the way she dictates. Change is threatening to her. She can stir up a lot of conflict when you try to develop new attitudes, because change is uncomfortable for her. Be prepared for your *parent* to strongly protest and make you feel guilty.

Your stabilizer is the *adult*. She is the one who can keep your mind on an even keel if she's been programmed with positive data—and that's your job right now. You'll want to program your *adult* for strong, positive attitudes that can override the whining cries of your *child* and the strong guilt-making commands of your *parent*.

The *adult* must also learn to console the *child* and reeducate the *parent*—no small job! (But it's possible through daily persistence and awareness.) You don't want to squash either one. You'll need all three to have a well-balanced personality. There are times when it's all right to have your *child* in command—when you want to have fun, to be a kid again. And you need your *parent* to keep you in line when temptations get in your way. The *parent* is your conscience.

The *adult* acts as a computer and sifts ideas through before making a decision. It's necessary to program your *adult* from this point on, so that all attitudes cause constructive, positive decisions that make you feel fabulous at forty-plus.[3]

There you have an extremely simplified picture of the conflicts that may be going on within you at mid-life. As if that's not enough, society threatens you further with its preoccupation with youth. It's no wonder we're tempted to look negatively at aging.

It would *almost* be easier to give in and begin a gradual decline rather than have to find your way through the maze of teenage idols, beautiful sex symbols, and deciphering what youth is all about. You've almost allowed your *parent* to convince you that youth is a time of life when skin is smooth and legs hop, skip, and jump.

On the other hand, if we're going to define youth in those illusive terms, then what are we going to call Sarah of the Old Testament days? She was ninety-one when she conceived a child—yet ageless. Her attitude was happy and vital, with a sense of humor too.

Like Sarah, some women never grow old. But others seem to be born old and stay that way all their lives. I remember plain Evelyn from high school. She was antiquated then and is now.

With her hair still pulled back severely in an unflattering bun and wearing colorless dowdy clothes, Evelyn clearly reflects her refusal to accept change. Through the years, her unbending ways have brought needless heartache.

If Evelyn could have developed an ageless attitude, some of her pain might have been avoided. Imagine how difficult Sarah's life would have been if she'd lost her sense of humor as well as the flexibility required to mother a new baby. By comparison, Evelyn's obsolete attitudes are bold thieves who rob her of life's pleasures.

How to Take Inventory of Your Negative Attitudes Toward Aging

What Evelyn needs is a mid-life checkup. Forty-plus is an appropriate time for anyone to take a mid-life check. Even your car, which is only a heap of cold, organized machinery, requires a periodic going-over if it's to operate properly. Surely, you deserve as much consideration.

Most of us are not aware our car has a problem until it begins sputtering. So it is with our minds. You may not realize you have unwholesome attitudes about aging until you hear yourself sputtering an ageist remark. It is imperative to check up on those negative attitudes if you are to develop an ageless focus and manage your life smoothly. Too many women carve their destinies from old-fashioned ideas, then wonder why they are so grouchy and cross.

Television's Archie Bunker comes to mind as we discuss unwholesome attitudes. Crusty ole Archie has ideas and attitudes that continually get him in trouble—yet he refuses to change his focus. Many women are like that. Here are some common remarks that will help you take inventory of your own attitudes.

The woman who is forty-plus and wants to feel fabulous *never* says things like:

"When I was young . . . ."

"I'm too old to . . . ."
"We're not getting any younger, you know . . . ."
"Sex! At my age?" (followed by a pathetic laugh)
"It doesn't make any difference at *my age* . . . ."
"No one notices *me* anymore . . . ."
"My mind doesn't work as well as it used to . . . ."

And an ageless attitude does *not* include these words:

I can't.
I'm not.
I shouldn't.
I wouldn't dare.
Why me?

Right now, go back and make some big red marks by the phrases that are part of your vocabulary. They indicate significant insight about your attitude toward aging.

Not only do words like that affect your attitude, they attract a negative response from people around you. They also attract negative-thinking people. Women of a feather negate together. On the other hand, an ageless attitude will automatically draw active-thinking people, who will further stimulate your ageless attitude.

As you ponder over your attitudes, think about how you feel right now at your present age. If you're honest with yourself, you'll no doubt discover a complexity of feelings—some positive, some negative. Chapter two will help you identify these feelings.

Keep a mental picture of an ageless woman before you. Don't lose sight of your goal. No objective can be reached unless the goal is clearly in sight at all times.

With your objective of an ageless attitude in sight, remember that you don't have to live your future in bondage to age. But it does take courage to make changes. You've taken an important step toward becoming an ageless woman when you decide you have the courage to be stronger than the opinion of your next-door neighbor or the outmoded opinion of society in general. "The *ageless woman* has the courage to turn her back on yesterday. She's the woman of today."[4]

Assignment: **The Inner You**

1. Think about and write how young you would be if you *did not* know your true age and *could not* see your body:

2. How do you honestly feel about your own age?

3. Can you admit you have conflicts about growing older? What are they?

4. Write at least five positive things about being the age you are:

Dream lofty dreams, and as you dream, so shall you become. Your Vision is the promise of what you shall one day be; your Ideal is the prophecy of what you shall at last unveil.

JAMES ALLEN

2

Moving Forward

... All things are possible to [her] who believes.[1]

In the last chapter you may have seen yourself in a new light, and now you want to make some changes. The question is: "How do I go about it, especially changing my attitude toward aging? I'm forty-plus and want to feel fabulous."

The first step is to break your pattern of negative thinking. You must remove the negative before the positive will take hold. Or, if you remember a popular song a few years back: "Ac-cent-tchu-ate the positive; E-lim-my-nate the negative, Don't mess with Mister Inbetween."

That's right! To be forty-plus and feeling fabulous, you must accentuate the positive. Eliminating the negative and all the stuff in between is going to be a slow process. I'll warn you now. Don't expect this to be an instant-magic program. It's not!

If you're looking for something easy, this isn't it.

If you're looking for something simple, you've found it.

The First Step: Breaking the Negative Thought Pattern

Before we go on, we need a clear definition of the word *attitude*. Webster has this to say: (1) the mental position with regard to a fact or state; (2) a feeling or emotion *toward* a fact or state; (3) the position of something in relation to a frame of reference. And Webster's definition of *mental* is also crucial: (1) occurring or experienced in the mind.[2]

Studying both definitions we clearly see that our *attitudes have been formed in our minds*. It is our own mental experience that has formed the frame of reference by which we make our judgments and set our standards.

To illustrate, when you see a gray-haired, wrinkled old man limp out of a bright-red sports car, you probably do a double take and wonder if he's going through an extended mid-life crisis.

BUT—if you see a beautiful young girl with long, blonde windblown hair, wearing tight jeans and a T-shirt to match, slinking out of a flashy sports car, you think the package all ties together the way it should. Old men don't belong in racy sports cars; young, seductive girls do. At dinner you're more likely to discuss the old man with these opening remarks: "You'll never believe what I saw today!"

This shows how you've conditioned your mind to accept and reject certain things. Your own experience has been the frame of reference by which you've made those judgments.

If you're forty-plus, you've had all those years to watch people grow older. Your mind has been busy registering the behavior of people over forty: the way they dress, wear their hair, how they talk, where they go, the decline in physical activity, the cars they drive, and many other subtle things. It's a blanket inventory. You don't consciously categorize, as I've done. But without your being aware, you've gathered plenty of data by your fortieth year. That's what sets the pattern for your aging process.

If you want to get started on developing an ageless attitude, the first thing you'll want to do is check out your own attitudes toward aging. Right now, sort through your own mental data

and with a bright-red pen, mark the words that best describe
your image of a woman over forty.

Hair:	Fashionable	Gray	Dowdy	Messy	Tight	Curly
	Short	Long				
Figure:	Fat	Sloppy	Square	Trim	Unflattering	
	Matronly					
Health:	Poor	Excellent	Good	Fair		
Dress:	Loose fitting	Fashionable	Drab	Unflattering		
Mind:	Stagnant	Growing	Poor	Good		

Physical Activity: None Some Very little Much

Interest in People: None Some Very little Much

Interest in Life: None Some Very little Much

General Attitude: Negative Positive Some of both
Tired Jaded

Productivity: None Some Much

Quality of Relationships: Poor Good Excellent

Social Life: None Very little Some
Much

Association With
  Women *Under* Forty: None Some Much Very little

Association With
  Men *Under* Forty: None Some Much Very little

Life-style: Sedentary Somewhat active
Extremely active

Now look over your check marks. If your answers don't indicate the highest potential in each category, consider your attitude toward aging as negative. Use this as a guide to help you
guard against developing that negative pattern of living.

As I've said, responding with a negative aging program is
NOT the way to be Forty-Plus and Feeling Fabulous. Secretly,
most of us fear changing from an active life to one of gradual
decline. Yet, until now, the options have been foggy.

Seeing the options can help remove the tension middle age
often brings. Many women (and men, too) become grouchy

and troublesome to their families and friends. This is a time of life when some try to cope by making radical changes in their lives. Those of both sexes eventually must reach a compromise within themselves. How aging is resolved either brings a new spirit of vitality and peacefulness or can increase the confusion and conflicts. Everyone wants a happy, peaceful life. Not all decisions lead there.

The good word is that you *can* have a happy, peaceful life. But are you willing to make changes in your attitude? I had to ask myself that question at a time of desperate need. Sometimes urgency makes change easier. The desire for change will be motivated by each woman's unique set of circumstances. The general problem we are working on in this book is building positive, ageless attitudes to cope with mid-life and create a productive future. However, each woman will have her individual problems to work out. That will be accomplished through releasing any negative blocks and building or strengthening the framework of faith in herself.

I had to make lots of changes in myself. They came through determination, perspiration, inspiration, and prayer. I did lots of praying. As I anchored my life in a deep belief in God, the changes gradually came. And God really kept his promise: "Whatever you ask in prayer, you will receive, if you have faith" (Matthew 21:22 RSV).

I claimed that promise from Matthew 21. I even wrote down the date to remind me—and I claimed His promise often. I didn't even know change was possible when I began that desperate but illuminating journey. Should you decide to claim that promise for yourself, don't expect drums and bugles to sound, though. God works quietly and subtly. He is such a smooth, efficient worker that if you aren't watching, you might miss some of His best accomplishments.

Some of you know what I've said is true. Some still have it to experience. Where you are right now doesn't matter. What does, is your willingness to let God make some wonderful changes in your life.

Just a word about prayer before I go on. When I first looked at myself and wanted change, I prayed. I must confess to you that I honestly did not expect answers to my prayers; they were more duty-prayers. My lukewarm, apathetic religious upbringing did nothing more than teach me to acknowledge God the Father up in Heaven—somewhere. He was distant and abstract, as He may be to you. It was a while before I knew a warm, loving, caring God. Here's how it happened.

God met me where I was. That happened to be in my backyard one sunny morning in Covina, California. Puttering around in my flower garden picking Shasta daisies, thoughts of God occupied my mind. While looking at a daisy, my relationship to God became simplified.

I saw the daisy petals as representing you, me, and everyone God has created. The center of the daisy represents God. Since each petal is connected to the Center, which is God, that showed me I have a direct line or connection to God. His Spirit is within me and is the connecting link. I am part of God. He is part of me. We are one, yet we are separate.

The connection makes it possible for me to have access to His intelligence, mental and physical strengths, wisdom, as well as the ability to make changes in my attitudes and life. Whatever I need that is within His constructive boundaries for my life is there for the asking. But I must believe I have it, after I ask.

That is where my faith plays a strong part in my life. If I ask, I receive. It's all up to me. Since God didn't create me to be a puppet whose strings He pulls, the moves are up to me. I like having that free choice. I also like knowing that God loves me enough to give me what it takes to grow and develop. As I've said, I'm only limited by my lack of faith—"According to your faith be it done to you."[3]

The message is simple, but many women make life difficult because they don't develop the faith that can bring a fabulous life at forty-plus or any age. God is *always* there.

I've found that God never changes in His love and concern

for me. His rules stay the same, too. *I can count on Him.* Even if I forget Him, He's still there reaching out to me—waiting for me to return.

One of the most important things I know about God is that He is constant. We live in a changing world. None of us know what tomorrow is going to bring to change our lives. But God is a stable, unchanging pillar in my life. I can count on that.

Not only did I find God to be an unshakable pillar, but through Him I learned to believe in myself. I learned to trust my own strengths and abilities. I found that I really could do all things through Christ who strengthens me.[4]

Every time I found doubt popping up, I'd repeat that verse to myself. I may have said it fifty times a day at first. One day I finally believed it!

Eliminating the Negative

The next thing we need to realize is that although some foods are delicious together, such as turkey and dressing, and potatoes and gravy, not so when it comes to negative and positive thoughts. Negative thoughts have no place in a mind that is trying to think positive. A successful blending of those two thought patterns is impossible. The negative thoughts must be swept away before it's possible to create a clean home for your precious, positive ageless attitudes.

Even in the New Testament times, Christ warned the people not to pour new wine into old wineskins, for the skin would burst and wine would spill as well as the skin destroyed. New wine must be poured into new wineskins so that both are preserved.[5]

Look at your mind as the wineskin that must be prepared for the exhilarating wine of positive thinking. Preparing your wineskin is going to take diligent, steady awareness.

I recall how it was when I decided to develop new attitudes, and became aware of my negative thoughts. I felt as though my wineskin would burst. It was a frightening feeling because I wasn't used to a multitude of negative thoughts such as came rushing to the surface at once.

Not knowing how to handle them, I asked my wise friend and pastor, Vic Dougherty. He advised me not to let them scare me, but simply to release one thought at a time. As I did so, I was quick to replace that space in my mind with a positive Bible verse.

Each time, I repeated a verse that built my faith in God and myself. It became easier as I practiced. I learned to like myself more and to be more accepting. My confidence also grew. That was a fringe benefit.

Awareness and release of those negative thoughts is always required in development of an ageless attitude. Turning loose of negative thoughts can be a struggle. They're like leeches and won't give up their hold on you without a fight.

Right now, think about the negative thoughts present in your life. Check off below the ones you have and add any that persist and flood your mind with conflict or anger—any thoughts which give you a lot of trouble.

Worry	Criticalness
Nonacceptance of growing older	Envy/Jealousy
Resentments	Self-pity

One way I found to help rid myself of unwanted thoughts was as Dr. Peale suggested. I'd go into the bathroom and mentally throw my destructive thoughts into the bowl—then I'd flush those thoughts away. In time, it became easier to release an unwanted thought. Eventually, I could simply release the thoughts by my own will.

I also learned to let Christ carry my burdens. Since I learned I could trust Him, I took Him up on that offer too. He says to come to Him if I'm tired and the burdens are too heavy to carry myself. All I have to do is take His yoke. He'll lift my problems and give me rest besides.[6]

Eventually, my mind no longer raced at eighty-five miles an

hour with worry and turbulence; it tuned down to a peaceful, normal speed and learned to relax.

Handling Fears

In addition to dealing with many negative thoughts, I had to uproot fears that had been so limiting. I learned to replace fear with faith in myself. I also found a trust in God that I didn't know was possible, as I made Christ a meaningful part of my life. I found through Him, truly, *all things are possible.* Remembering to keep His rules for living at the center of my thoughts helps to keep everything else in proper perspective.

No trouble is too big to handle; no emotion too unbalanced. Fears do not get out of hand. And now at mid-life, age and physical changes will not cause me undue stress, because my life is not built on how my body looks, although that is important to me also.

Mid-life can aggravate fears and create misery. I was brought up with fear. I was afraid of the dark, afraid of strangers, afraid of my father's stern discipline, and afraid of God. I was afraid of life. Before I found out God is a gentle, loving, forgiving Father, fear dominated my life.

Fears can be blown out of proportion. As an example, the incident I'm going to share may seem ridiculous to you and wouldn't even cause your heart to skip a beat. But to me, it was a real fear and caused dread and anxiety.

I was in my early twenties and had just learned to drive. Near the center of town were two sets of railroad tracks spaced several yards apart so that two or three cars could wait between them if necessary. One day I was driving over the tracks when the old-fashioned control gates closed on either side—something I had dreaded. There I was, sandwiched between two sets of railroad tracks. Trains rushed past me on either side. I was forced to come face to face with fear! I wasn't hurt, of course. And it wasn't nearly as bad as I had allowed my fears to imagine.

It wasn't until after my study of *The Power of Positive Thinking* that I learned coming face to face with fear is the best way to overcome it. I also learned "perfect love casts out fear."[7]

There isn't much in this life that can be sidestepped. And that includes fear. But sometimes we have to realize that we actually enjoy our fears. We'd rather be afraid and go into a shell, or hide from reality, than face up to our fears.

Every time I begin to enjoy a fear, I remember this biblical warning: "For the thing that I fear comes upon me, and what I dread befalls me."[8]

I thought I had learned my lesson, when my anxiety level rose again a couple of years ago. My husband was born in New Hampshire, and skiing is second nature to him. After an absence from the slopes of several years, he decided to start swooshing again.

Being a southern California beach type, I knew I'd better learn to ski if I planned to keep up with my husband. I signed up for weekday classes—four weeks before our scheduled ski trip to the French-Italian Alps. I boarded the bus with all my new gear and headed for Mount Hood with fifty other women.

My friend Jani, who is an accomplished skier, was also taking lessons (advanced). She knew I was afraid to ride the chair lift, so decided to teach me ahead of my scheduled lesson. She was patient and sympathetic. But she became so involved with my fear of the chair, that as we both stood there waiting for it to come from behind, with Jani explaining how I should position myself, and I concentrating on her instructions, we both forgot the most important thing—the chair!

In Jani's attempt to teach me, she'd accidentally stepped out of the chair's range. The chair came abruptly, bumped me from behind, and knocked me half into it—as Jani stood to the side watching. The blow jarred me, and my ski poles planted themselves in the snow below.

I wiggled my body back into the chair. But I was on the lift by myself, going the mile—a ten-minute ride—for the very first time! A-l-o-n-e! I feared heights. I was moving up the hill. The chair began swaying in the wind. Below me I could see deep holes in the snow. Had skiers fallen out of their chairs?

It was a long way down there. How was I going to get off the chair? When would I get off?

My heart was pounding so loudly I could hardly hear the wind howling around my swinging chair. I tried deep breathing to calm myself. Then I remembered the familiar verse that has carried me through many situations: "I can do all things through Christ who strengthens me." I thanked God for that strength, then called to the skier in the chair several feet ahead of me. He shouted back: "Just keep your ski tips up when you pass the big basket, then put them down flat. Use your chair to push off and ski down."

"Oh, sure," I thought. At the halfway point was the first off-ramp. I had a choice. I opted to stay on and survey the landing carefully so I'd know what to expect when the second exit time came. As the chair approached the ramp, I saw the sign, PRE-PARE TO GET OFF—then I saw the huge spider's web, woven to catch falling skiers, with a sign warning, KEEP TIPS UP.

Trembling, I cautiously slid to the edge of my chair, holding on as though death were tugging at my arm. Tips up! Whewww—didn't fall into the basket! Skis flat—now push away—and go-o-o-o.

When Jani arrived several chairs later, I was there in an up-right position, smiling and waiting. I had conquered my fear.

Thank God for faith in Him and in my own ability. He gave me confidence again when I needed it. He never lets me down *when I remember to turn to Him.*

I know it's not always as simple as I've made it sound. Some-times a person's fears can be too strong. For some people the misery can seem better than change. Familiarity can give a person a false sense of security: a feeling of all-rightness and confidence, says Cecil Osborne. Through many decades of counseling, Dr. Osborne has seen numerous people resist changes that could bring them relief from stress, ill health, and decomposing relationships. Fear holds them back.

At forty-plus, the fear of adopting new attitudes can stifle life instead of open new doors. There is fear of failure, fear of people, and fear of rejection, to name a few. All these fears can subconsciously block entry to the development of an ageless attitude and can keep you from feeling fabulous.

In addition, you won't feel fabulous if you allow your fears to run out of control. Fears aggravated by worry and feeling insecure can also create illness.[9]

There are many reasons then for taking Dr. Peale's advice to empty your mind of fears. You'll be able to sleep better if you empty your mind daily before retiring. The last five minutes before going to sleep are of extraordinary importance; in that brief period the mind is most receptive to suggestion. The mind tends to absorb the last ideas you entertain in waking consciousness.[10]

Right now would be a good time to think about your own fears. Check off any of the fears that are hindering your ageless attitude:

Fear of:		
Dying	Change	Getting ill
High places	Being alone	Other people
What other people think	Traveling	Being rejected
	Getting older	The dark
Driving	The water	Making decisions

Jot down others as you think of them:

Fear-filled thoughts can clog the mind and stop the flow of mental and spiritual power. I have used Dr. Peale's flush method of emptying my mind of fear and know it works. After I empty my mind, I say something like: "God is now filling my mind with courage, with peace, with calm assurance. God is now protecting me from all harm. God is now guiding me to right decisions. God will see me through this situation."[11]

Fear is a powerful emotion. But faith is stronger and can overcome fear. My faith in God has grown strong, but I also have faith in myself now. I want you to have the same faith in yourself. You'll enjoy knowing you can do just about anything you set out to do. Don't allow fear to keep you from developing an ageless attitude and feeling fabulous.

Fear can manifest itself as a lack of confidence, too, and keep you from taking the step toward your vital ageless attitude. Dr. Peale says the greatest aid to eliminating an inferiority complex, or self-doubt, is to fill your mind to overflowing with faith. He also suggests building your faith and trusting God more and more each day, as I have. It takes time, but you can develop a tremendous faith in God that will give you a humble, yet soundly realistic, faith in yourself.[12] Matthew wrote the same thing several different ways: "According to your faith be it done to you," and "If you have faith . . . nothing will be impossible to you!"[13]

We'll leave Matthew and progress on our journey to becoming Forty-Plus and Feeling Fabulous. Most of us don't pay too much attention to our own words, but we should. Become aware of the words you say. Whenever you catch yourself saying things like, "I'm too old to . . . ," replace that negative attitude with a positive statement of faith. One of my favorite verses, as I've said before, is: "I can do all things in him who strengthens me."[14]

Then, whenever you catch yourself making a decision based solely on your age, flush that away and immediately make a decision based on more substantial reasoning. Think *ageless*. Reinforce your growing belief in yourself and that *age is no barrier to abundant living*. You're developing an ageless attitude. Write that on your mirror with lipstick so you can see it often.

While you're changing, if someone ridicules your new ageless attitude or if you become discouraged, instead of slipping back into your old pattern of thinking, train your mind to automatically shift into positive. Expect stumbling blocks.

And now, as I conclude this chapter, I have shared what a large part my religious beliefs have played in shaping my ageless attitudes. I don't know what your background is. You may have been brought up in a conservative, fundamental home, or you may have little or no understanding of Christianity or the Bible. What I've tried to do here is give you some principles that are true no matter what your relationship to God is at this point.

The first step to becoming ageless is being aware of negative attitudes. Then you must get rid of your negative thoughts and start to live according to faith. My own experience has been that faith in God and the teachings of the Bible have been powerful influences in developing a solid foundation for my commitment to change from negative thinking to positive.

And it's never a case of I'm too old, but *I can do.*

Assignment: **Moving Forward**

1. Increase your faith in yourself and in God daily.
2. Be constantly alert for negative attitudes. Every night before going to bed and in the morning before getting up, empty your mind of every negative thought in your awareness.
3. After emptying your mind, immediately fill it with positive, life-building statements of faith or inspiration. Use this chapter, the Bible or other sources of inspiration.
4. Daily, visualize yourself as a positive, energetic, vital woman who has an ageless attitude and is Forty-Plus and Feeling Fabulous.

Those who are quite satisfied sit still and do nothing; those who are not quite satisfied are the sole benefactors of the world.

LANDOR

3

Making the Transition to an Ageless Attitude

Love is patient and kind. . . .[1]

Let's take a look at what we've done so far in our effort to develop an ageless attitude.

We have learned to recognize negative attitudes toward aging. We've seen the importance of having a sound foundation, which I believe is essential to changing an attitude.

And as I've shown you, I have been able to lay that foundation in my life, through knowing God and replacing negative-thought trends with positive scripture.

Now we are ready to begin making the transition. Building a lasting, unshakable foundation will take constant perseverance on your part. Making the transition will be a *daily effort*—not a one-time shot. Transition will be a vital part of your growth process. Remember, no one ever arrives—we just keep striving for the perfection that requires a lifetime effort.

One of the vehicles we will use to help achieve an ageless attitude is the use of list making. Perhaps it's already part of your daily planning; it is mine. I'd be lost without that method of organized thinking. Many executives use and attribute their success to list making.

Throughout this book, I will ask you to make lists. Some of them will be easier than others. They will all help you get your life organized and help you move toward feeling more fabulous.

One way to feel more fabulous is to learn to discard negative attitudes. Discarding those attitudes can be pretty discouraging sometimes. I want to caution you about that right now. Think back to when your children were babies. Remember how patient you were while they were learning to walk?

Back in chapter one, I described one way of seeing the human personality as a *parent, child,* and *adult.* You will recall the *parent* is the authority; and the *child* demands attention. Here is your chance to be a better *parent* to the *child* within by allowing your *parent* to give the kindness, love, and patience every growing *child* needs.

One of the ways I learned to be patient with myself was through one verse that reminds me: "Love is patient and kind."[2] Because I feel patience is so important to your growth, I'll be reminding you to love yourself and be patient many times throughout this chapter.

A Focus on Your Positive Qualities

Because many of us have never learned to love ourselves properly, we fail to see our positive qualities. It's hard to admit the good things about ourselves. Early training taught us not to brag. We think it's sinful to be aware of our good qualities, and when someone compliments us, we squirm instead of accepting it graciously.

Christ taught: Love your neighbor as yourself.[3] Yes, loving self is one of life's necessary laws. But unless we learn to love ourselves first, there'll be no love for our husband, kids, *or* next-door neighbor. Self-love is not to be confused with conceit, which is a cover-up for feelings of inferiority. That kind of love also separates us from those we'd like to love.

Right now, I want you to make your first list. Jot down the qualities you like about yourself:

1.   8.

2.   9.

3.   10.

4.   11.

5.   12.

6.   13.

7.   14.

If you found that a difficult assignment, here is some help. Your list might contain some of these things.

I have good health.	I am intelligent.
I am a worthy person.	God loves me.
I'm an efficient homemaker.	I am a faithful wife.
I have the ability to love.	I like people.
I'm attractive.	Children like me.
I have a pretty smile.	I'm kind to animals.
I'm an excellent cook.	I'm a good seamstress.
I'm a loyal American.	I am honest.
I am creative.	I am well-groomed.

Try to list at least ten, if you can. I know this is a difficult assignment. In the Yokefellow groups I've led, people respond to this request with shuddering hesitation. Take this opportunity to think about the many good things that comprise the very special package called YOU. Demand the freedom to see yourself in a positive way.

I know you're thinking someone might say you're conceited or without humility if you "toot your attributes" publicly. Consequently, you haven't even tooted them privately.

If you have found writing complimentary things about yourself to be uncomfortable, begin with the most simple compliment you can give yourself. I'm going to help you sort through the many qualities and talents you have taken for granted.

If you've been a homemaker (not a housewife, please), you have countless abilities. Experience has made you an expert at the duties you shrug off as "nothing." You've been running a mini-corporation from the kitchen sink, without ever realizing it. Can you visualize yourself as an important executive? A VIP?

And now, will the real executive please stand up?

As you read on, with a bright-red felt pen, make some BIG checks by all the things you know you do well or have experience in. Be generous but honest. These positive qualities will nourish you as you chip away at the negative ones later on.

Your talents are many:

Washing, ironing, cooking, sewing, mending, cleaning;

Plumber, electrician, painter;

Landscaper, interior decorator;

Nurse, doctor, counselor, therapist;

Teacher's aide, home economist, home manager, social secretary, accountant, purchasing agent;

Sunday-school teacher, choir member.

(Only an executive could manage so much!)

Your ability to love is broad:

Husband, children, family, friends, and stray puppy dogs.

You're not only a wife, but:

A gracious hostess, a silent business partner, a compatible traveling companion, a reliable sounding board, a good listener, and a darn good sex partner.

In addition, you may:

Be attractive, have a pretty face, a nice body, beautiful hair, or a perfectly shaped nose.

Have flawless olive skin like Sophia Loren, or a peaches-and-cream complexion like Scarlett O'Hara.

Possess intelligence, academic degrees, talent in crafts, pottery, writing, art—the list is endless.

Now congratulate yourself for a job well-done! Not many of us who have stayed home to raise families and run households have seen ourselves as executives. But we've earned the title and didn't even have to go into the marketplace to fight for it.

In a sense, what you're doing is similar to writing your own eulogy while you're still alive and can bask in it. I've always felt it is a terrible waste to wait until people die to give them praise. I'll have my flowers and compliments now, please!

All the Things You Don't Like About Yourself but Were Afraid to Tell

I hope you have really given a lot of effort to finding your positive qualities. You'll need them to keep you in balance. It's usually not a good idea to focus on the negative unless you have something to offset it. But it is necessary to deal with the negative side of our personalities if we are to progress to an ageless attitude.

And so, it's time to make a list of all the things you don't like about yourself but have been afraid to tell anyone—even yourself!

We're going to get right into it. The best way to get wet is to jump into the water. You'll not only be working on negative attitudes, but physical qualities you dislike about yourself, as well.

This time, use a black pencil with a good eraser on the end. Begin making your list of negative qualities, both mental and physical. After you've made your list and begun working on removing a specific quality, you'll be able to erase it from the negative list. Then you can add a new one to the positive attributes. Personally, I like to keep the lists as I've written them so I can look over from time to time. Then I can see where I've been. That lets me see growth. I get excited when I can see progress in my life, as you will.

Are you thinking about your negative attitudes? Okay, take a deep breath, grit your teeth, take pencil in hand, get on your mark, get set—now wriiiiiiite!

1.	9.
2.	10.
3.	11.
4.	12.
5.	13.
6.	14.
7.	15.
8.	

You probably didn't come up with too many at this first try, so here is some help to trigger your thoughts:

It's too late to change my attitudes.	I can't.
I'm afraid.	My mind is going.
I don't care.	If only I'd . . .
Everything from the ankles up sags.	Why does it happen to me?

I don't have anything to do with my life.

I'm not young anymore.

Who would want me?

I can't trust God.

I don't have enough money to . . .

No one likes me.

If only . . .

I'm not attractive anymore.

I can't learn anything at my age.

I'm too old to . . .

I'm too old to start exercising.

I feel sorry for myself.

I'm stupid.

I'm afraid of . . .

I don't care how I look.

I'm too fat.

I'm too old to get married again.

I'm too old to enjoy sex.

I overeat.

I don't like myself much.

I smoke too much.

I drink too much.

I hate my nose.

I'm scared to change.

My hair is drab.

My teeth look awful.

I feel old.

List as many as you can right now. You can always add to your list as you become more aware of your negative attitudes. Your awareness should grow keener as you focus on attitudes. This is a painful process, but do try to be honest with yourself. No one else is going to see your list unless you show them.

If your mind gets stubborn, as mine sometimes does, I find this little verse helpful: "Search me, O God, and know my heart! Try me and know my thoughts!"[4]

Searching does take honesty, as I've mentioned before. Attitudes are harder to find than the physical imperfections we all have to live with. But let's face it. There are some physical changes you won't be able to make. I quit wasting energy on them a long time ago and came to grips with those imperfections I could do something about. At seventeen, after I went to work, I had my teeth straightened and eliminated what I considered a major problem. I've learned ways to make myself more attractive with becoming hairstyles, makeup, and fashionable clothing. Exercise helps, too.

Fretting over your less-desirable qualities is a waste of time because it doesn't change anything. It does magnify the problem and create a negative disposition, though.

Many people are bothered by a nose that is oddly shaped or too large. Part of my husband's charm is his shapely Jimmy Durante nose. He hated his nose as a child. But as he grew older, he learned to accept and love his nose. He even makes jokes about it. He has turned his nose into a large asset for his personality. That up-front honesty is one of the qualities I love about him.

If you have a nose problem, you have two options. One is acceptance; the other is plastic surgery. My youngest sister, Judy, had her Italian nose reshaped and feels 100 percent better about herself. She also became a Christian at about the same time and that might have had something to do with her new self-esteem. I am reminded that James said you can't just tell people to " 'Go in peace, be warmed and filled,' without giving them the things needed for the body. . . ."[5]

Of course, having your nose reshaped is costly and time-consuming. I find the best way to accept myself in any problem area is to tell God about it. I ask Him to take away whatever attitude I'm hassling with. Then I replace the nagging in my mind with something positive about myself and from the Bible. Then I thank God for releasing me from my burden.

Why is it we tend to forget who created us and become critical of our design? This is the verse that reminds me the Great Creator designed me: "You made all the delicate, inner parts of my body, and knit them together in my mother's womb. Thank you for making me so wonderfully complex! It is amazing to think about. Your workmanship is marvelous—and how well I know it."[6]

With the bombardment of top fashion models on major-magazine covers and beautiful women on television commercials, we have a tendency to compare ourselves and come out on the short end. If we had the same makeup artists and hair designers as those women, we'd have more of a chance to look perfect, too. And remember, models only look that way while they're being photographed! After that, many of them look like ordinary people.

Later on we'll discuss exercising. That's the only way to trim away parts of the body that have managed to become unruly through overeating or living too sedentary a life.

Right now, don't become discouraged! Concentrate on changing one negative attitude and making one body improvement at a time. Don't tackle them all at once; you'll get discouraged and quit. It's not going to be a quick, overnight process. Remember how many years it's taken to accumulate them all. Great accomplishments take time. Even gifted Michelangelo knew he could not create his great masterpieces in a day; sometimes it took years.

Again, I'm going to remind you to *love yourself* and *be kind to yourself.* You, too, are a great masterpiece—worthy of all the effort you'll channel into sculpturing an ageless attitude so you can be Forty-Plus and Feeling Fabulous.

Formulas for Change

"Are there any easy formulas for change? If so, I hope Ruby gives me some," you may say. Remember what I said in chapter two? If you're looking for something easy, this isn't it. If you're looking for something simple, you've found it.

I'll be giving you some simple formulas, but they all require persistence. After my high-school graduation, I worked for an attorney as an apprentice secretary. Right off, he dictated a proverb I've carried in my wallet for over thirty years. It says:

> The thing that we persist in doing
> comes easy in that we persist in doing it.

That little saying may not mean much to you at first glance. I didn't catch the full significance until many years later when the card was worn around the edges. Simply stated: The more you do a thing (no matter what it is) the easier that thing becomes, because—you keep doing the same thing. As you keep doing it, it becomes easier to do.

Applied to bad attitudes, which become habit patterns of thinking, you can see why they continue on and become so difficult to break.

Applied to newly acquired ageless attitudes, this positive statement reinforces the hope that the attitude will become easier as it is used, developed, and used again. Eventually, the new thought pattern of ageless thinking will become strongly reinforced in your mind. This attitude will then become a permanent part of your living pattern—just as the unwanted negative attitude was.

For example, I can remember that I used to think I was not good in sports. Because of my mother's blinding fear that I might hurt myself, she never allowed me to skate, ride a bike, or even swim. Her fear became mine, and I developed an "I can't" attitude that not only affected my confidence but my coordination in athletics as well.

A few years ago a friend asked me to play tennis. Instead of allowing my negative "I can't" attitude to control my decision, I began playing. So far I've made excellent progress. I still have a long way to go, but I am changing my attitude toward my ability to play. Now I'm in the habit of playing tennis and trying other sports too.

> The thing that we persist in doing
> comes easy in that we persist in doing it.

When you want to change, you can even pretend at first. In *The Art of Understanding Yourself* Dr. Cecil Osborne explains the James-Lange theory for change: "If we check or change the expression of an emotion, we thereby change the emotion itself. Put another way, if we 'act as if' we feel a given way, in time our feelings catch up with our actions."[7]

Dr. Osborne relates his own experience when as a young minister in his first church, he decided to apply the James-Lange theory. He says:

> When calling in a home, I found myself wanting to talk about the church. I was quite uninterested in the seemingly trivial details of the lives of the people whom I visited. I was a poor conversationalist, with a strong dislike for small talk. This was a distinct handicap, for when calling on members (of the church) I found *they* wanted to talk about things that interested them—their children, a new piece of furniture, the little incidents of the day.
>
> Upon entering a home I began deliberately to pay attention to the children, to notice details, such as the pictures on the mantel, antiques—everything that seemed of importance to the family, and to comment on these things. I even tried to enjoy the cats which shed hair on my dark suit. At first I felt uncomfortable and hypocritical: after all, I wasn't genuinely interested in these details. I wanted to get down to the really "important" matters, such as their relationship to God. . . . But in time I began to enjoy my experiment and felt less hypocritical and insincere. Before long I was discovering a genuine interest in the details of their lives . . . because they were important to the people on whom I was calling.
>
> Ultimately it became second nature. I ceased to think of myself solely as a budding young prophet possessed of transcendent truth. . . . I came to be genuinely interested in people and in anything which mattered to them. It was not simply a new technique but a new self-image. I began to "see" myself as a different kind of person and to act in harmony with my new image.[8]

Today Dr. Osborne is past seventy-five. He is a living example of an ageless attitude. He looks as vital as he did when I first met him over twenty years ago. I'm so glad he made a decision to change his self-image and develop a genuine interest in people. That decision to change made him a happier, more successful, man. But it also allowed him to touch and change the lives of thousands of people, including mine, through Yokefellows and the Burlingame Counseling Center in Burlingame, California.

Dr. Osborne travels and lectures throughout the world. Besides taking an active part in the two centers, he continues to write books on how to have a better life—because he keeps finding new ways for life to become more abundant.*

The 21-Day Plan

Developing a more abundant life is going to take plenty of persistence. Dr. Maxwell Maltz, author of the excellent book *Psycho-Cybernetics,* says it requires a minimum of about 21 days for an old mental image to dissolve and a new one to jell. Dr. Maltz makes this suggestion:

> During these 21 days do not argue intellectually with the ideas presented, do not debate with yourself as to whether they will work or not. Perform the exercises, even if they seem impractical to you. Persist in playing your new role, in thinking of yourself in new terms, even if you seem to yourself to be somewhat hypocritical in doing so, and even if the new self-image feels a little uncomfortable or "unnatural."[9]

How do you make this 21-day plan work for you? Simply by using it as a springboard for changing negative attitudes to positive. Since it takes at least 21 days to establish a habit, that is exactly what you will be doing—establishing a new habit. It will be a constructive one that trains you to reinforce or add positive attitudes and get rid of the negatives.

---

* Cecil G. Osborne is author of: *The Art of Getting Along with People, The Art of Becoming a Whole Person, The Art of Understanding Yourself, The Art of Learning to Love Yourself, The Art of Understanding Your Mate,* and others. The Yokefellow center is located at 19 Park Road, Burlingame, California 94010.

Let's redefine our long-term goals: *Your goal is to be Forty-Plus and Feeling Fabulous by developing an ageless attitude that allows you to think positive and to live a life based on your vitality, not your age.*

However, all of that is not going to happen in 21 days. You'll simply be laying the groundwork so that your goal can be achieved over the next several weeks or months, depending on your commitment. Remember, life is a continuous growing process; don't grow impatient. Change takes time.

That's what my friend Jackie found out. At forty-seven her old habits of thinking negatively about growing older were so well ingrained that Jackie thought developing an ageless attitude and feeling fabulous were beyond her reach. She thought it was too late! But we spent several long lunch hours pouring over her inability or unwillingness to let go of these attitudes that were obviously curbing her vitality.

First of all, Jackie was unhappy with her useless attitudes toward age. She wasn't a slob by any means, but there was definitely room for improvement. The upper half of her body showed gravity pull, and she edged dangerously close to matronly dressing to cover the bulges. She hated the way she looked and the feeling of growing older. But like so many other women, she'd bought and accepted the whole negative concept of getting old from society. Finally, Jackie decided she had nothing to lose by trying out the 21-day plan for change.

This is the way Jackie attacked her problem: First she made a self-commitment. She knew that was important if she was sincere about changing. She pictured herself with an ageless attitude and a new image—a slimmer, more active woman. Then she made a list: first, of her positive qualities; then her negative ones to change. She knew that more would pop up as she grew in her awareness of herself; she'd add those to the list, too. She was realistic and didn't expect to see all the negatives at once. Neither did she want to!

Then, every morning and every night and during the day

when she was driving, pressing a skirt, or cooking dinner, Jackie concentrated on flushing away the negative attitudes. Then she'd quickly replace them with positive reinforcement, such as her good qualities or a positive verse from the Bible.

She'd ask herself questions like: What am I thinking that could be more constructive? Do I base my decisions on my age? How do I allow my age to control my life destructively?

Jackie learned something about negative attitudes: People are not disturbed by the things that happen (including aging) but by *their opinion* of the things that happen.[10]

When Jackie planned an activity, she asked herself if she was capable of doing something more challenging. Would there be people of all ages—not just her own? At luncheons or meetings she'd try to determine if the conversations would be on gossip, housework and kids, or if there would be mind-expanding discussion to learn from. Slowly, Jackie began to create a growing kind of environment for herself.

Jackie had one problem that troubled her deeply. She had never learned to swim and longed to enjoy the water like others she watched. After her physical checkup, her doctor told her to "go for it" and go for it she did. But it wasn't that simple! This is where she was really going to test the 21-day plan. She outlined her problem:

Problem:	Can't swim.
My negative attitudes:	I can't swim. I'm scared of the water. I'm too old to learn. I look awful in a swimsuit.
What I'll tell myself for 21 days: (Developing the new attitudes)	I want to learn to swim. I'll learn to swim so I won't be afraid of the water. I want to play in and enjoy the water.

	I'll lose weight and tone my body so I can look good in a swimsuit. I'll read up on swimming now.
Taking the action after 21 days: (Putting the new attitude into action)	I *can* learn to swim. I'll buy a one-piece swimsuit that makes me look as trim as possible now. I'll sign up for swim lessons. I'll sign up for exercise and diet classes. I'll lose weight and tone body.

Well, you can see that Jackie killed several negatives with one positive. There was also an unexpected bonus. Jackie's husband started swimming again, and now they swim together once a week. "We're both feeling better," Jackie beams. She has a special glow and an excitement about life that was missing before.

"One of the really neat things about being Forty-Plus and Feeling Fabulous," says Jackie, "is that my husband's attitude is changing too." Yes, Glen is a changed man. Why not? He is lying beside an ageless woman every night; an ageless woman sits across the dinner table; and he, too, is feeling more alive and vital—a reflection of his wife's new ageless attitude.

Change is not easy! Developing an ongoing ageless attitude such as Jackie's is not a 21-day process. It will take a lifetime to develop, as I've said before.

You can do the same thing. This is the way to begin: Daily, hold a mental picture of yourself as you'd like to be. Keeping that picture in your mind is important because it allows your subconscious mind also to act toward meeting the goal. A woman always acts, feels, and performs in accordance with what she *imagines* to be true about herself and her environment.[11]

Daily, take at least five minutes in the evening before retiring and five minutes in the morning when you are completely relaxed to again remind yourself to accentuate the positive, eliminate the negative. Then be conscious of your attitudes all day. Remember to *be patient* with yourself if you happen to fall short one day. Changing is a *daily* building process. Don't let one failure discourage you. If you made a decision based on your age yesterday, use that failure as a reminder to go forward!

During these 21 days, combine all the other processes we have discussed so far to help shift from negative attitudes to an ageless-attitude focus.

You may not see evidence of anything happening at first. But be assured that your subconscious mind is busy at work effecting changes—if you're consciously doing your part.

When I'm in a specific process of change, it helps me to remember God created me in His own image. If I were creating something, I would not deliberately engineer my product to fail. I can't believe God created me to go around with a hangdog expression, being miserable, afraid of life, or feeling that life is over at forty-plus.[12]

You know, it's funny how tiny events stick in your mind for a lifetime. I was in the third grade, standing by a water fountain at school. A little friend asked: "Do you think you're pretty?" I giggled. With embarrassment I indicated a quick no.

"Then you've insulted God!" she smirked.

And it's true. "God don't make no junk." As you change your attitudes to positive, remember—it *is* a compliment to your Maker when He sees you succeed and use to the fullest, the abilities and talents He gave you.

The 21-day plan is one way to reprogram your mind with positive, ageless thinking. After that, it's an *everyday effort,* as I've said before. But what you build today builds on tomorrow and the next day and on into your entire lifetime.

During this time of changing, let me emphasize again—be patient with yourself. If you slip, forgive yourself. It's not the end. Pat yourself on the back for having tried and for the progress you have made. Then go on from there.

Assignment: **Making the Transition**

1. Begin the 21-day plan today. Choose one specific item from the list of negative attitudes you prepared earlier. It's important to remember to work on only *one item at a time* for 21 days so you don't become discouraged. Now fill in the following outline to begin the first attitude change. (Refer back to Jackie's outline if you need help.)

   Problem:

   My negative attitude: (How it affects me)

   What I'll tell myself for 21 days: (Positive attitude)

   How I'll take the action after 21 days: (Putting the positive attitude into action)

2. Read over the positive qualities you have already listed. Add any new ones that may have come to mind. Fortify your mind with those positive qualities each day for 21 days to help develop the habit of positive thinking.
3. Again, check over your list of negative qualities. Add to the list any new ones that may have surfaced. Do not dwell on these, but arrange in the order in which you plan to change them.
4. Practice releasing your negative thoughts by using the flush method. Then replace them with these thoughts:
   ... If God is for us, who is against us?[13]
   I can do all things in him who strengthens me.[14]
   ... the kingdom of God is in the midst of you.[15]
5. Be patient and loving with yourself. Do not condemn yourself for failure.

Part II

Conquering the Myths in Menopause

4

Avoiding Menopause Panic

A cheerful heart is a good medicine, but a downcast spirit dries up the bones.[1]

In chapter three we talked about changes and how to start to make those changes in your life. At this time it would be good to think about a major change in your life that will be occurring whether you want it to or not—menopause! How can you keep your ageless attitude when menopause arrives?

One of the ways is to understand what menopause is, what it can do to you, and what you can do about it. Too many women blame their mid-life crisis on "the change." Yet, menopause is just an innocent bystander, doing the job God programmed it to do: make you sterile.

The word *menopause* has a negative connotation in our society. I wish this could be a talking book so you would hear the negative tone when women say, "the change."

Since that's not possible, read this letter I received from a friend that clearly reflects the possible emotional and physical turmoil menopause can bring to the woman who is not prepared for the inevitable mid-life change.

65

Dear Ruby:

You asked what's the matter with me. Not only am I going through the menopause, but I'm a "has been." I used to be a girl. Now I'm forty-eight. I bitterly resent the changes these years have brought. I hate the aging process and the social attitudes that relegate people my age to the "old fogey" category.

Middle age is a lonely, terrifying time. My children are building their own lives. My women friends are engrossed in their own physical and emotional discomforts.

My husband dismisses my behavior as menopausal. He either doesn't realize or won't admit, that he, too, is undergoing subtle changes.

More and more I feel middle age is a shameful thing—and I *am* ashamed of my moods, my attitudes, and my appearance.

If I'm tired, I'm a party-poop. If I eat what I like, I'm a glutton. If I smoke, I'll die of cancer (but not soon enough). If I lose my temper—or cry—I'm emotional, or worse, having hot flashes. If I stay up late at night, I'm trying to avoid sex. If I complain about being tired or picking up after everyone, I'm a nag.

If I sleep-in, I'm slothful. It's an unwritten rule I must never let anyone think, even for a moment, that I'm feeling sorry for myself.

Ever try putting eye makeup on while you're wearing bifocals?

Menopause is frustrating and I'm fed up with it. Having hot flashes, getting soaking wet and having to remove and replace bedclothes all night is not funny and I'd rather not be teased about it.

If I don't feel like sex, I'd rather feel free to say so—and have my husband sympathetic toward my feelings occassionally—without having to feel all the guilt of the archenemy of manhood.

It hurts a lot never to feel pretty anymore; it's difficult to be responsive. Being old and ugly has its compensations?

The loveliest thing about today is that tomorrow I'll be my sweet, lovable self again.

Miserably,
MICHELLE

Tomorrow did come for Michelle. But the scars of her menopause and mid-life changes remain. It isn't easy to repair the damage that has been caused because you and your husband have not understood what has happened. We'll be looking at some of the things Michelle didn't know, in this and the following chapters.

Many women feel the same isolation and bewilderment as Michelle because they are afraid to talk about menopause and what they are experiencing. Myths and fears make menopause mysterious instead of another phase of development. Let me encourage you not to be shy about talking—first, with your husband. He needs to understand what is happening to you.

Then talk with other women about menopause. This subject has been locked in the closet far too long. When you do talk about menopause, you'll be surprised at the quick, eager responses. Women are anxious to talk about their problems as long as they feel sure their symptoms are no different from yours. Sharing is one good form of therapy.

Paradoxically, for a subject that is extremely important to our lives, education has been scant. During menopause, not knowing about the symptoms and the way mid-life can bring panic is a serious problem. "You will know the truth, and the truth will make you free"[2] is not only wise, but essential, at menopause.

If someone asked you what you would like to know about menopause, how would you respond?

In a survey, an overwhelming majority of women made no response at all. A few women replied they had never thought about it, and one woman asked, "Is it true that women go crazy while going through menopause?"[3]

The answer is NO! Going crazy because of menopause is a myth. In this chapter we are going to take a long, hard look at menopause and its dangers. It's not to alarm you or make you dread menopause (if you haven't already experienced it). Preventative medicine is still the best remedy for staying mentally and physically healthy.

For menopause, preventative medicine adds up to self-education. You'll save yourself endless frustration and unhappiness during an already difficult time of life by learning all you can before entering the change.

And don't be afraid to say *menopause*. Repeat it over and over until it feels comfortable to say. Menopause is not a dirty word.

What Is Menopause?

Menopause is a stopping of menstruation. Hooray! No more periods. This distinct hormonal change leads to the inability to have children. While menopause itself is a short happening, it's the adjustment to your changing body that takes time.

According to many doctors, 20 percent of all women experience no problems during menopause. Ten to 15 percent have severe symptoms, including nervous breakdown or severe depression, and the other 65 to 70 percent experience a few symptoms in varying degrees. These include the following:

1. Tendency to gain weight with a redistribution of fat
2. Tiredness
3. Sleeplessness
4. Temporary lessening of desire for sex
5. Depression, mild to severe
6. Vaginitis, itching, irritation
7. Headaches
8. Leg cramps
9. Dizziness
10. Heart palpitations
11. Aches and pains
12. Opening leading to the bladder and part of bladder becomes thinner, sometimes making it difficult to empty the bladder (can cause bladder infections).
13. Gradual thinning and drying of vaginal tissues due to estrogen reduction (can make sexual intercourse painful unless lubricant is used)

14. Loss of fatty tissues from the external vaginal folds, which gradually become smaller as do the internal folds; vaginal walls may become relaxed from loss of muscle tone
15. Hot flashes: wavelike sensations of heat that move up to the chest and to the head, frequently followed by profuse perspiration. Flashes may last a few seconds or as long as thirty minutes to an hour and are more frequent and disturbing at night.
16. Breasts have tendency to become smaller and flabbier from decrease in fat cells.
17. Psychological changes, including anxiety, increased tension, mood depression, and irritability
18. Osteoporosis (bone loss)[4, 5]

That's the bad news. But it's really not as grim as it seems. You're not going to experience all the symptoms at once—and you may not experience any of them, other than the stopping of your monthly flow. But it's helpful to know the signs so they won't interfere with your being Forty-Plus and Feeling Fabulous.

Besides trying to keep your ageless attitude, the important thing is to be prepared. But for some reason, I wasn't even thinking about menopause when it sneaked up on me. Happily remarried for almost three years and occupied with college, menopause didn't even cross my mind. Even with a background in psychology and a better-than-average understanding of myself, it caught me unaware.

Three months passed before I recognized the symptoms. Since I'd had a hysterectomy ten years before, there were no erratic periods to flag me. The first warning was extreme fatigue. I couldn't get rested. Then concentration became difficult. I had several near auto accidents because my thinking was clouded, but God kept His hand on my steering wheel and controlled my brake.

Finally, the thought hit me that I might be starting the

change of life. I called my doctor. He could see the change in me as soon as I walked through his door. My sprightly step was gone. My swollen eyes no longer sparkled. I cried all over my doctor: "Am I really going through the change?"

Yes! However, there was good news, too. There is medical help to get us through the "bad" times. We don't have to roll in the snow like our grandmothers did to cool off during a hot flash!

As a word of encouragement, let me say that I have experienced very few symptoms from that list I gave you. I have not had hot flashes or many of the feelings Michelle shared in her letter. The persisting symptoms have been vaginitis, bladder infections, and the need for a lubricant during sexual intercourse. Low-grade depression was a minor problem when estrogen ran low, but my body has adjusted to the diminishing supply, so having the blahs is rare for me.

What Causes These Problems?

Why in the world must women experience so many problems during menopause? There is a simple answer. It's lack of estrogen. Menopause is the time when our bodies are adjusting to a diminishing supply of the estrogen those healthy, plump ovaries have been working so hard to produce. But now the ovaries are going into retirement. They are gradually shrinking. That means the amount of estrogen being supplied to your bloodstream decreases.

It all starts during puberty, when the sex hormones (including estrogen) that have been in minute supply since birth begin active production. For a woman, the production of estrogen is cyclical—each cycle lasting about one month. Each cycle is caused by the gradual build-up of sex hormones, which peak during the interval when an egg leaves the ovaries. After ovulation, sex-hormone production begins to taper off and reaches its lowest point just as menstruation begins.

During puberty and again during menopause, there is a discreet change in the levels of sex hormones circulating in the female bloodstream. The pubertal change reflects the switchover from low to high hormonal levels. The menopausal change is the result of a switch from the high levels to the lower premenstrual levels.

Physical, emotional, and even behavioral changes can be tied to the cyclic pattern of sex-hormone activity and to the distinct changes of hormone supply between one phase of life and the next.[6]

As an example, you may have experienced premenstrual blues or postnatal depression; and now at menopause, you also may experience some psychological and physical disorders.

Coming to your rescue are the adrenal glands. At this time they often step up production of estrogen and help your body adjust gradually to the changes taking place during menopause.

Your physical and mental health will determine how beneficial your adrenal glands can be to you, however. If they are exhausted because of mental or physical stress or nutritional abuses, they cannot produce the buffer of estrogen your body needs. That is when your body may reflect a lack of estrogen and you may be forty-plus, but not feeling too fabulous. It's important to be aware of what's happening to you so you don't become overwhelmed by menopause.[7]

Sonya is a woman who did get overwhelmed by menopause. Unfortunately, when we make wrong decisions, they not only affect and hurt our own lives, but those people we love as well. For Sonya, there was a husband, two children, a Siamese cat, and their lovely Cape Cod home in New England.

To the onlooker they seemed no different from the average American family with typical problems. All appeared well and healthy—all except Sonya's husband the morning he arrived at work weary, drawn, and white. Sonya wanted a divorce not only from her husband, but from all her responsibilities—including her aged parents, who lived with them. She offered no reason for the change.

However, there had been subtle hints. Sonya's shiny blonde hair turned to harsh henna. Conservative clothing gave way to sexier, more revealing styles. A new urgency developed in her manner and movements. These were the outer signs of the discontentment stirring deep inside.

Since Sonya couldn't handle the problems of daily living that every normal family has, she simply made an exit. Midlife panic! She felt she had sacrificed everything and could no longer cope with it. The pressure of growing older clouded her vision. Perhaps Sonya's perspective might have been different if she'd only realized she was feeling some common frustrations of mid-life. Her conflicts were compounded by an inability to cope because of her diminishing estrogen supply.

Sonya is just one of many unfortunate women who enter mid-life with blinders. Psychological changes turned love for her husband into resentment and eventual divorce. All too late, Sonya learned those feelings were temporary. She'd made the biggest mistake of her life and regretted it.

Menopause can affect a woman's coping ability. Too often destructive attitudes develop that are far too strong. Those attitudes generate destructive courage that would be better used working out problems and setting constructive goals.

Another radical change in personality occurred in a woman we'll call Terri. A youthful, forty-plus-eleven, Terri's slender body and chic blonde hair created an image that was perfect for her responsible job in a large San Francisco firm.

But suddenly Terri made an abrupt change in her conservative life-style. Leaving her husband, she moved into an apartment to be "single." She collected a few male friends and adopted an anything-anytime philosophy. The sudden change was completely out of character for Terri. Friends and acquaintances just shook their heads and whispered: "Terri must be going through the change."

Terri was indeed going through the change. Hormone imbalance during menopause can bring about abrupt changes such as Terri's. Although the examples of Sonya and Terri are extreme, they do happen. The divorce rate is exceptionally high during mid-life because changes are difficult to handle and even more difficult to understand.

It wasn't necessary for Sonya or Terri to fight her way through menopause and end up only with battle scars. And it isn't for you, either. Getting proper medical help right away and trying to keep your ageless attitude will help you cope with defeating frustrations menopause may bring.

When Can I Expect Menopause?

You can lessen your frustration by knowing what to look for. The erratic menstrual flow will signal the beginning of menopause and will alert you that more changes are on their way, physically and emotionally.

However, women who have had a hysterectomy prior to menopause will not have that signal. That makes knowing what to anticipate even more critical.

Menopause is difficult to pinpoint because it doesn't come at the same age for every woman. There is a definite association between the beginning of menstruation and the arrival of menopause. Girls with an early puberty usually have a potentially long reproductive career and a late menopause.

Menstruation at the age of ten, for instance, would bring menopause around the age of fifty to fifty-two. However, if your period began at the age of twenty, unfair as it may seem, you might experience menopause as early as thirty to thirty-two.[8]

My period began at the age of eleven and menopause arrived at forty-seven. But I was thirty-six when my doctor first wondered if I might be entering the change. We had moved from California to Washington. With my roots deeply implanted in California, the move caused me extreme stress. But after a few months, the feelings of depression and the blahs vanished. It was a false alarm!

When menopause does arrive, remember, it is only one more

change in a life full of changes. This is the last hormonal shift and the final stage (hallelujah) in your physical sexual development. Being free from the worry of pregnancy is one more reason to celebrate being Forty-Plus and Feeling Fabulous. But how you react to menopause will probably be similar to how you reacted to your other sexual changes.

As I make the changes in my own life, there is a verse that speaks to me even in menopause: "How wonderful to be wise, to understand things, to be able to analyze them and interpret them. Wisdom lights up a man's [woman's] face, softening its hardness."[9] When I really hear those words, I want to examine the changes that seem unnatural or are out of character for me, because I want to keep within God's constructive boundaries for my life.

And now, before going on to the next chapter, which will tell you more about menopause and give you the pros and cons of estrogen therapy, let's pause for an assignment.

Assignment: **Avoiding Menopause Panic**

1. Reread Michelle's letter. With a red pen check off any of the feelings you identify with.
2. Go back to the list of symptoms and check off those you may be experiencing.
3. Read this chapter to your husband and discuss menopause. Then talk about your feelings and physical discomforts.
4. If you answer yes to any of the following questions, you should seek medical help right away.
   a. Do you have hot flashes?
   b. Are the hot flashes frequent?
   c. Do you have vaginal dryness?
   d. Is the vaginal dryness causing pain during intercourse?
   e. Do you suffer from depression?

It is possible to be youthful at any age, except when you're young.

SAMUEL VAUGHAN

5

Getting Through Menopause—The Pros and Cons of Estrogen

For wisdom is better than jewels. . . .[1]

There is help for menopause. One of the basic ways is with estrogen therapy. While estrogen supplements do a terrific job of combating that long list of symptoms you read about in chapter four, it does have some side effects. One of them is the danger of cancer.

The possible connection between estrogen therapy and cancer is an *extremely controversial subject,* and I don't even pretend to give you advice in one direction or another. I only want to give you the facts so you can weigh them and make your own decisions. Read everything you can find on this subject.

Discuss the pros and cons of estrogen therapy with a doctor whose judgment you trust. Then you'll have to make your own decision on whether or not you will risk the possible long-term effects of estrogen. I prayed for wisdom and direction, then proceeded cautiously.

This has been my experience. Again, I want to emphasize

that I'm not saying it was the right decision or the one you should make. But it helped me glide through menopause with a minimum of emotional upsets or physical discomforts. My major discomfort has been wrapped up in the estrogen-therapy scare.

Whether or not to take estrogen therapy was my dilemma! It was an extremely serious decision for me because of my family's strong history of cancer; both my parents had the dreaded disease and lost the battle. Mom, a beautiful, vital fifty-five, was enjoying her empty nest and grandchildren when the doctor discovered cancer in her breast. Even though a radical mastectomy was performed, cancer spread throughout her body within five years.

You may wonder, as I, whether or not my mother had taken estrogen therapy. It's hard to admit I don't know the answer. Yet, this is a typical attitude about menopause—women don't talk about it. And since I didn't know anything about menopause in those years, there was nothing to ask.

It's tragic and sad when daughters know nothing of what is happening in their middle-aged mothers' lives, physically or emotionally—particularly at menopause, when emotional support is desperately needed.

Because of breast cancer on the maternal side of my family, I had even more reason to be apprehensive about estrogen therapy, but I decided to go ahead.

When I went for treatment, my doctor warned me of the immediate side effects as well as the long-term dangers. He asked me to keep a diary of physical discomforts from estrogen therapy and report them regularly. I experienced chills and slight nausea at first, until my body adjusted to the new estrogen. Those side effects usually lasted only a few hours on the day I received the injection.

Not everyone takes estrogen by injection as I did. My doctor chose that method as a means of keeping a close watch, rather than prescribing estrogen in pill form that is taken daily. Conscientiously, each week, my doctor gave me small dosages of estrogen.

Cautiously, he watched to be sure it agreed with my body chemistry and to be sure there were no harmful side effects. After several weeks, the doctor increased dosage to five milligrams of estrogen. For the first year, my treatments were from six to eight weeks apart, or whenever I needed estrogen. I tried to prolong the interval between treatments whenever possible.

"Patients come for treatment more often when they are under stress, or some unpleasantness is going on in their lives," my doctor warned.

Those first injections of estrogen were water-base in nature. Later I changed to a longer-lasting oil-base estrogen. However, the oil-base has a disadvantage: If your body reacts to it, you must live with the effects until the estrogen wears off. My side effects were chills (unlike chills from being cold), with a slight nausea similar to morning sickness. I ate soda crackers every morning for three weeks. I'd had no morning sickness during my two pregnancies, but here it was during menopause!

After that, we switched back to a water-base estrogen. In my third year of menopause, I needed only two injections spaced many months apart. Now, at fifty-one, I don't anticipate needing estrogen any longer—most of the discomforts are gone.

However, some of the medical specialists I have talked with recommend that menopausal and postmenopausal women continue taking minimal dosages of estrogen for the prevention of osteoporosis (bone loss, which can cause the hip fractures so common in the later years). We will discuss this later in the chapter.

Even though I had estrogen therapy, I was never completely peaceful about it. I continued to read everything relating to estrogen and cancer. In a college health course I prepared my term paper on the subject. Everything I read emphasized the dangers of estrogen therapy.

You'll want to know what these dangers are, so I will briefly list them. Your doctor can explain them in detail.

The Potential Dangers of Estrogen

Short term:
1. Nausea and vomiting
2. Breast tenderness or enlargement
3. Excess fluid retention
4. May cause depression
5. Allergic rash

Long term:
1. Endometrial cancer (cancer of the lining of the uterus). The woman who has had a hysterectomy is not exposed to this danger.
2. Breast cancer
3. Tumors: cervix, vagina, liver
4. Gall bladder disease
5. Abnormal blood clotting[2]

Every pharmaceutical company encloses detailed information about the dangers of estrogen with every prescription; it should be read and understood. Again, I emphatically urge you to do your own research. Your library will have many of the books on my suggested reading list at the end of this book. If you're near a university, their medical journals will give you the latest studies. Research is ongoing.

If reading is a must, then routine breast exams are a *must-must!* Since I've always had lumpy, cystic breasts (not uncommon), a new lump is hard to detect. When I'm in the shower, I find soapy skin makes routine breast exams easier. Examine yourself at least once a week. About one out of eleven women will develop breast cancer. At present, it is the leading cause of cancer deaths in women. But breast cancer caught early has an 85 percent chance of cure.[3]

To guard against cancer, my doctor routinely checked for changes or new lumps before giving me an injection of estrogen. Since it's easier for you to recognize those changes or additional lumps in your breasts, you should work as a team. Always ask your doctor to verify what you've found. It doesn't pay to take chances with your health.

These are the warning signals: breast changes that persist, such as lumps, thickening, swelling, puckering, dimpling, skin irritation, distortion or scaliness of nipples, nipple discharge, pain, or tenderness.[4]

In addition to routine checks, mammograms (breast X rays) are recommended every year for women over fifty; less often for those under fifty.

However, X rays are not without cancerous effects on your body. Research is now being done in diaphanography (DPG), non-X-ray ultra-sound equipment. As a light scans the breast, images and shadows flash onto a TV-type screen for a specialist to interpret. Unfortunately, there are not many in use as yet. Ask your doctor about this new way to detect breast cancer.

If you don't have a family history of cancer, your doctor may want to use other methods of estrogen therapy. Ointments and suppositories are two options, but the most popular is the pill form. It is estimated that 10 million American women take supplemental estrogen in pill form alone.

Whichever form of estrogen therapy is for you, self-education will increase your ability to talk with your doctor intelligently. You'll want to know what's going *into* your body as well as what's going *on* in your body.

These are some additional things you'll want to ask your doctor if you're having estrogen by injection:

Brand name of estrogen

Oil-base or water-base

How many milligrams? (You should never have more than five.)

Is it synthetic or animal estrogen?
  Which is best and why?

Side effects: long-term and short-term

You'll want to carry the name and dosage in your wallet. If you're on vacation or out of town, you'll have the correct information, and a new doctor treating you won't have to guess what you've been taking or how much. It's silly to spoil a vacation because you're having hot flashes and don't know what kind of estrogen agrees with you.

While you're having estrogen therapy, your doctor may recommend physical exams every three months. You should have exams and a Pap test every six months at least. However, with the increased danger of breast and uterine cancer, the quarterly exams are advisable.

For those at high risk of developing cancer, other hormones such as progesterone and androgen have also been found to be useful to some degree. You'll want to ask your doctor about the alternatives to estrogen therapy.

The Dangers of Not Taking Estrogen

In addition to the dangers of taking estrogen, you've got to think about the possible effects of *not* having this important hormone. If you don't take estrogen, you may be passing up help to combat the bone disease that is common in aging women—osteoporosis.

Osteoporosis is a subject that gets little attention but should be of major concern to us. It is the loss of mineral calcium from the bones and is generally more prevalent in women.

Calcium is what gives bones (and teeth) their strength and hardness, and there is more of it in the body than any other mineral. Osteoporosis comes from a negative calcium balance, which means the body is losing more calcium than it is taking in and retaining. The bones lose bulk and density and become more porous and brittle.[5]

Research shows that bone loss is related to advancing age, but there is now substantial evidence showing that bone loss in women is related to the diminishing supply of estrogen that begins in menopause.[6]

In an interview with Dr. Sheldon Spielman, a noted Portland, Oregon, obstetrician and gynecologist, he expressed these concerns about treating women for bone disease:

> In order to prevent osteoporosis, estrogen must be given within a couple years of the onset of menopause and maintained for life. If a woman waits too long to take estrogen, the bones will go through an irreversible change and the calcium loss will continue in spite of estrogen therapy.
>
> Although estrogen therapy does relieve menopausal symptoms, its *primary purpose* should be for the prevention of bone loss.
>
> However, long-term estrogen treatment for bone loss is not recommended for women who have a family history of cancer or for women who have *not* had a hysterectomy.
>
> But, for the woman who *has* a strong history of osteoporosis in her family, *but no breast cancer,* there is an alternative. It might be advisable for her to have a hysterectomy in order to take life-long estrogen. This would eliminate the high risk of cancer of the uterus as well as osteoporosis.
>
> For the woman who *does not* have a strong heredity factor of osteoporosis, there is an alternative to estrogen therapy. Maintaining normal body weight, a trim figure, and good muscle tone and keeping physically active and having a well-balanced diet might be infinitely safer than to be on estrogen for life.

Again, whether or not to have estrogen therapy for life is best decided with your own doctor. But, as I've indicated before, the final decision can only be made by you. More and more women are seeking second opinions before undergoing surgery or other treatments—and wisely so.

Hysterectomy and Oophorectomy

When women reach forty-plus, they sometimes have to have a hysterectomy. Many women fear that a hysterectomy will cause them instant menopause, but that does not happen unless you also have an oophorectomy.

With over 8 million women in the United States having had a hysterectomy, it has become a household word. However, many women do not realize that a hysterectomy does not include the removal of ovaries. A hysterectomy is the surgical process in which the uterus, or some part of it, is removed.

The medical term for the removal of ovaries (or ovary) is *oophorectomy*. Since the ovaries are the main producers of estrogen, you can see the importance of keeping them as long as possible. Even one ovary can do the job if it becomes necessary to have the other removed.

Ovaries are removed surgically because of disease or nonfunction or a malignant tumor. But the decision to remove your ovaries should be arrived at with your doctor only after careful consideration. If your ovaries are to be removed, you should know about it before surgery. You'll be asked to sign papers to that effect in the hospital. Read that permission form carefully so you'll know exactly what your surgery will include.

The removal of both ovaries will bring an instant menopause to a woman of any age.

The woman who has her ovaries removed before her normal menopause will no longer produce estrogen, except for the tiny amount made outside her ovaries. You can see then, to take away a woman's estrogen supply is a serious step because of the drastic changes it will produce in her body.

Long-term estrogen replacement can be given, but your own estrogen is always best—not only because it is made by you and for you, but because your body regulates it according to your day-to-day needs.

If it becomes necessary to have a hysterectomy and an oophorectomy, after a day or two you will experience the menopausal symptoms of hot flashes, heavy sweats, and possibly some of the other discomforts we've already talked about. Even women who have already gone through menopause may experience those symptoms if their body was still making estrogen before their surgery.

To relieve the menopausal discomforts after surgery, estrogen-replacement therapy may be started while the patient is still hospitalized.

Unlike the gradual diminishing of estrogen during normal menopause, the sudden stopping of natural estrogen because of surgery is more difficult for the body to adjust to.[7] One woman who had a hysterectomy and an oophorectomy has a difficult time maintaining mental equilibrium at times because estrogen replacement doesn't always perform as well as her own would. Sometimes she's irritable and cross. She cries easily. Other times, she's sweet, easy to get along with, and copes well.

Right now, finding the right doctor may be a worse problem than menopause. Dr. Howard Judd, from UCLA, says that until recently menopause was largely neglected—except by women who entered it. "We're a society which deals with men and youth. Start talking about the problems of older women and people turn off. Since the condition is seldom life-threatening, many doctors have tended to discount the importance of the menopause and dismiss it as an inevitable—and unpreventable—part of the aging process."[8]

Because of this discouraging prevailing attitude, be sure you know the attitude of the doctor treating you. Does he understand what menopause is all about? Is he sympathetic to the problems of menopause?

If your doctor ignores your problem and tells you it will pass, better find a new doctor, quick! Talk to other women to find out which doctors are tuned in to menopausal problems.

Insist on your right to be heard and treated properly.

After you've found the right doctor and begin having treatment, you can again give your full attention to developing your ageless attitude. Medical help will make this stage of your life better so you can enjoy being forty-plus.

Assignment: **Getting Through Menopause**

1. List your family's medical history. Was there cancer or osteoporosis on the maternal side of your family? Give this information to your doctor.

2. Make a list of questions you want to ask your doctor. When you make an appointment, ask for the last hour on his calendar. That will give you more time to talk, and he won't feel rushed. Take the list of questions with you so you won't forget any of the things you want to know or discuss. Tell your doctor you have a list of things you'd like to discuss with him, so he won't dash off before you've had a chance to talk with him. Invite your husband to sit in on the discussion.

3. Begin your weekly breast exams. If you find any of the cancer warning signs, report them to your doctor immediately.

4. If you are already on estrogen therapy and are still having menopausal symptoms, ask your doctor to try a different kind of estrogen.

5. Read and discuss this chapter with your husband.

Part III

Beauty Is Skin Deep and Then Some

6

Feeling Fabulous With Your Body

*Do you not know that you are God's temple
and that God's Spirit dwells in you?*[1]

In the first five chapters you have worked very hard—
stretching your mind. It has wanted to rebel at times, just as
your body does when you think about stretching it—which just
happens to be the next challenge awaiting you. Please don't
turn away before you see how easy it's going to be.

I know you're probably tired of seeing the many-splendored
exercise and diet programs beckoning on every national magazine cover. They keep appearing—and women keep buying
them. We all know diet and exercise are important—but apparently just not important enough to do much about them—
for Americans are truly in bad shape! If you don't believe me,
just people watch for fifteen minutes.

Not all of us are in real bad shape. Some of us are just lean-
ing in that direction. A small roll of excess flesh seems to come
from nowhere and glues itself above the waistline, making it a
bit difficult to look trim and tailored with our clothes neatly
tucked in. Some of us have quit wearing short-sleeved blouses
because of fatty arms and flabby underarm skin. And some
even hesitate squirming into a one-piece skirted swimsuit be-

cause there's no longer a way to conceal what has been happening to our bodies.

Ho hum!

Is that what middle age is all about? How can I be forty-plus and feel fabulous when I'm beginning to look "flabulous?"

That was the question Andrea must have been asking herself. The other morning I hurried by her house to drop off a book I'd borrowed. As I was about to knock on the back door, I could hear some moaning and groaning in the backyard, so I peeked around the corner of the house. As I swung the little white gate open and started up the stone path to her patio, there was exercise-determined Andrea. She was dressed in baggy red shorts, a large white sweatshirt, and a pair of red tennis shoes with fluffy balls peeking over the heels. Andrea's strenuous exercise was producing enough blood, sweat, and tears to water the entire garden.

Andrea looked up, paused, and made an attempt to smile. "Oh, Ruby, I'm sure glad it's you! I've never worked so hard in my life. I keep thinking I need to keep myself up and be active. But every time I try to get some kind of exercise program going, I get frustrated."

"You never told me you were into this kind of thing, Andrea," I commented.

"I'm not, really. This is the fifth time this month I've started. I actually hate exercising—it's an absolute effort—I'd almost rather take a whipping. At first, I throw myself into it. Then I get so sore that I stop. And it's hard to get started again. I just wish someone would invent an electronic computer that could program flab away!"

Andrea is no different from many of us. Few of us are athletic jocks who can hardly wait to work out each day. I do have one exceptional friend; Connie can be seen jogging through downtown Portland every lunch hour—preparing for one twenty-six-mile marathon after another. But she's the only woman I know who's that motivated.

The rest of us need something easier, less demanding. That's why Hyman Jampol, author of *The Weekend Athlete's Way to a Pain Free Monday,* has developed a program based on stretching, rather than torturous, sweat-producing exercises. Director of the Beverly Palms Rehabilitation Hospital in Los Angeles, he has found that by stretching, you can get rid of pains and prevent future injury—simply by maintaining flexibility and preparing your body for exertion. The aim of stretching is to condition the connective tissue that binds together your bones, muscles, and other movable body parts.[2]

Even with the availability of less-demanding health programs, people don't take time for their bodies. The average woman is involved in school, employment, or housework, and none of her activities provide an adequate overall movement of the total body.

That is why I have developed this easy fitness program. It will take only a few minutes a day of your time. Not only that, the program will tie into some of your present daily routines. Because of this, the new exercises can easily become habitual.

The important part of the program is your commitment—the same as it was in the first five chapters. The disciplines you have learned will help you habituate this positive action as well.

Why Be Fit?

Besides the reasons Mr. Jampol gives for keeping physically fit, here are more:

1. To withstand fatigue for longer periods
2. To develop a stronger and more efficient heart
3. To develop mental alertness
4. To reduce nervous tension
5. To eliminate sagging, flabby tummies
6. To strengthen stomach muscles to eliminate back pain
7. To develop stronger lungs
8. To feel fabulous at forty-plus

Keeping in mind the many reasons for committing yourself to this program, let's get started.

Lung Power

I know you wake up in the morning, smile, lean over, and kiss your husband good morning, tell him you love him, then jump out of bed with all the enthusiasm of a kid going fishing on a warm summer's day. (Well, it's a nice thought, anyway!)

But before you jump out of bed, take a moment to increase your lung power. Most people use only the upper part of their lungs, so their breathing is shallow. The purpose of this exercise is to use your whole lung capacity. This exercise has helped increase my wind capacity while jogging.

- Empty all air from your lungs by slowly *exhaling* through your nose. As you exhale, pull in your abdominal walls to assist in complete emptying of air.
- *Inhale* through your nose. Begin breathing slowly and at the same time slowly push out the abdominal area by using your abdominal muscles. (This forces air into the lower part of your lungs.)
- While you continue to *inhale,* push out the stomach slightly and expand your chest as far as possible. As you inhale, raise the shoulders as high as possible, to allow the air to enter the high parts of your lungs. Hold as long as comfortable.
- Repeat.

Remember to begin slowly and do only a couple the first time. It will take a while to coordinate the abdominal positions with your breathing. Some people experience light-headed feelings at first because they are used to shallow breathing.

With all the fresh, new air breathed deeply into your lungs, you're ready to jump out of bed, if your husband hasn't already pushed you out. It would be wise to let him know about the breathing exercises in advance, so he doesn't think you're having an asthmatic attack.

Now, run to the bathroom, pick up your toothbrush, apply toothpaste; then go at those teeth and gums gently.

Lower-Body Toner

While you're brushing your teeth, you're going to stretch those toes, feet, lower-leg muscles and abdomen, and tighten the buttocks.

- Pull in your tummy muscles as though protecting yourself from a right hand by Sugar Ray Leonard.
- Rise up on your toes, both feet together, and stretch as high as you can, as though you were wearing extremely high-heeled shoes. Stretch until your calf muscles feel very firm.
- Lower your feet to a flat-footed position.
- Repeat slowly while you brush your teeth, working up to ten the first day. As you get used to the stretch, hold your stomach muscles firm, as well as your buttocks tight. Slowly build up to thirty-five.

Remember to take your time and not push yourself. You're developing a pattern of stretching, not competing in an athletic competition.

The Loofah Rub

While you're showering, give yourself a loofah rub. A loofah is a rough-textured sponge we're going to use for a friction rub. These sponges can be purchased in department or health-food stores and come in various shapes. I'm told no self-respecting Frenchwoman would be caught without her loofah! It creates smooth skin, they say. I soap mine and use it to keep my heels, knees, and elbows from getting rough. It's also good for getting rid of dead, dry skin.

Towel Twist

After you've showered, the next stretch is accomplished with the use of your bath towel, as you're drying yourself.

I hope your bathroom is larger than a tiny cubicle, because you'll need lots of elbow room.

- As you dry your back, use the towel in the same way a shoe-shine person polishing shoes uses the cloth. Using both hands, hold your towel at each end and rub the towel across the back of your body, starting with your neck, and working down across the buttocks. Put lots of vigorous movement into your body.

If you're forty-plus, you may remember a dance called the Twist, popular back in the sixties. This exercise resembles the movements of that dance.

The Rollaway

After you've dried off your body, you'll want to work a bit more on your waistline. This stretch is done in a simple, circular waist movement.

- Stand with your feet about six inches apart, placing your hands on your hips. Slowly bend the upper half of your body forward to a comfortable position. Then slowly rotate your body to the left and around, in a complete circle, at the level where you feel the muscles stretching.
- Repeat this complete circular motion five complete revolutions.
- Then revolve to the right for five more circular motions.
- Increase the amount at your own speed.

Heart Throb

Your heart probably gets the least amount of attention, yet it should get prime time. It only takes a minute or two of your time to insure a healthy, strong heart. My doctor recommends running up and down the stairs a couple of times a day. You can run to the kitchen for your first cup of morning coffee.

Jogging in place for a few minutes each day can also exercise your heart.

If you have no stairway in your home but work where there is one, use it instead of the elevator. Consciously think of ways to increase your body's activity. Walk whenever you can.

Sensual Woman

While you're having that first cup of coffee, sit back and think about the day ahead. While you're doing that, you'll be doing the sensual-woman exercise. It's a very important one; yet it can be done anytime, anywhere, without anyone's knowing about it.

As we grow older, especially at forty-plus, the inner muscles of the vagina relax and need to be strengthened. Tightening these muscles does two things: It makes sexual intercourse more enjoyable both to your husband and to you. And it can help control involuntary urination, which is sometimes common during the forty-plus years. With the decrease of estrogen, the tissues that were once strong, elastic, and flexible become less tight.[3]

To tighten these muscles is simple.

- Tighten the vaginal muscles by squeezing as though you were trying hard to hold back urine.
- Tighten and hold to the count of ten. Then relax. Do five times. Or you can do one, several times during each day. After a while, it will become a habit. If you can tie the habit into another routine thing you do, it can trigger the exercise into action. For instance, if you drink coffee throughout the day, let the coffee remind you to begin the vaginal exercise. Driving is another good time to squeeze those muscles.

Headstrong

While you're watching TV, you can become headstrong. Actually, it's a head-and-neck rotation.

- Sit with your back straight (preferably in a chair). Look straight ahead. Slowly turn your head to the left as far as you can without discomfort. (Try to line up the tip of your nose with the tip of your shoulder, only *don't* bring your shoulder to your chin.)
- Repeat to the right.
- You may feel some tightness or discomfort at first. The idea is to *stretch those muscles gently and slowly* until the day comes when you no longer feel any pain. Then keep doing the stretches daily so you don't become stiff again.[4]

Slim Chin

The double chin is not uncommon at forty-plus in American women. It may be true that French women never get double chins because their language forces the use of those facial muscles. But we must exercise to maintain a slim chin. And it needs to be done in privacy, for it isn't a facial gesture you'll want to share.

During the day, you'll no doubt need to visit the bathroom several times. Put that time to double duty. Look up to the ceiling, close your eyes, and do the following as long as you are there:

- Pretend to chew gum exaggeratedly by opening your mouth to its widest and closing it tightly.
- Pucker up for an exaggerated kiss, then push into a large smile, moving those facial muscles as fast and wide as possible.

As you can see, snatching tiny bits of time here and there is what is going to make your body feel more fabulous. This stretching program doesn't take a great deal of time, so you should feel quite optimistic about committing yourself to this routine.

When day is over and your thoughts turn to rest, use the time just before retiring to continue making your body feel more fabulous.

Wrinkle Discourager

Even removing your makeup can be a beneficial exercise. Massage the skin upward while applying your makeup remover (or soap) and during its removal. If you use night cream, again massage the cream into your skin in upward strokes, away from gravity pull. The same rule follows for applying your foundation in the morning.

Bosom Lifter

One of the places gravity pull becomes obvious is in our bustline. But breasts need not sag. Just a few minutes of exercise every night will keep them firm and work wonders for your arms as well. Skin has a tendency to become loose on the inner upper-arm area that seldom is exercised. This motion will help all the problems we just mentioned:

- With your arms extended forward beyond your bosom, bend your elbows and grasp the opposite wrist tightly beyond the wristbone, with each hand. Use a push-pull movement.
- As you push the skin toward the elbow, if you're doing it correctly, you will see the arm and breast muscles all move. Hold for three seconds, relax, and repeat. Begin with ten if it's easy for you. If not, work up to it slowly. I do this thirty times nightly.

More for the Bosom

After you finish the bosom lifter, stand where you won't hit anything with your arms.

- Starting with your arms down by your sides, extend them forward, at least breast high. Clench your fists and in a quick, swinging motion swing arms backward as far as they will go.
- Then bring arms forward and release fists on the way.
- Repeat.
- Do as many as is comfortable the first night. Work up to thirty-five.

This movement helps tighten sagging underarm skin and tightens chest muscles.

Knee Raising

You can do this one while watching the evening news, if you have a TV in your bedroom. Otherwise, do it in the bathroom right after you've removed your makeup.

- Stand straight and keep your feet together, with your arms at your sides.
- Raise your left knee as high as possible, trying to touch your chest. Pull your leg against your body with your hands.
- Repeat with right knee.
- Do this stretch slowly and only a few times the first day, increasing the number daily. Stretch! See how long it takes you to reach forty-plus.

Back Flexibility

For the last two exercises, you can actually crawl into bed. With two pillows under your head, stretch out on your bed.

- With your left leg straight on the bed, bend your right leg and slowly bring your right knee toward your head, grasping it with both hands. When your knee has come up as far as it will go, lift your head and try to touch your forehead to your knee.
- Repeat with the left leg.[5]

More Back Flexibility

After this exercise, you can turn off the light and go to sleep.

- With your head still propped up on two pillows, lying on your bed, bring one knee up toward your head, then the other, grasping the front of each knee with your hands.
- Pull both knees toward your shoulders. Next bring your head up between your knees and try to touch your knees to your temples.[6]

Remember, this is a stretching program, basically. It is not going to take off excess weight. You may want to sign up for a physical-fitness course and get yourself in shape. But first, I recommend using Hyman Jampol's method of stretching to condition your body. And again, the doctor should give you the go-ahead before you begin any physical-exertion program.

Weight Control

If you do decide to commit yourself to a physical fitness program, you definitely want to learn about weight control. The major purpose of weight control is to reduce the amount of fat on the body and to increase the amount of muscle. Rather than weight control, it might better be called fat control.

This is what happens: Excess energy is stored as body fat. When fat is not used, it becomes excess fat. Besides looking unsightly, extra weight places a burden on your heart and muscles. (However, excess energy used up by a regular exercise program leaves no extra fat to burden and misshape your body.) For example, if you eat food containing 3,000 calories and use only 2,600 of them in your daily activity, the remaining 400 calories are stored in your body.[7]

Every time you accumulate about 3,500 unused calories, you'll notice an extra pound when you stand on the scales. One extra pound doesn't sound like much in itself, but when you think of it in terms of one a year for forty years, that's forty extra pounds you could be carrying around. And this is one time forty-plus is *not* fabulous.

When you keep active, you burn off the extra calories; it's that simple.

I find I can eat almost anything I desire and maintain a healthy body weight as long as I exercise (and don't eat hot-fudge sundaes too often).

Below is a chart showing ideal weight according to height, and the approximate calorie intake needed per day to maintain that weight (based on moderate activity).

Height	Weight (Normal Range)	Daily Maintenance Calories	Present Calorie Intake	Present Weight
WOMEN (20 years and older)				
5'0"	100–118	1500–1770		
5'1"	104–121	1560–1815		
5'2"	107–125	1605–1875		
5'3"	110–128	1650–1920		
5'4"	113–132	1695–1980		
5'5"	116–135	1740–2025		
5'6"	120–139	1800–2085		
5'7"	123–142	1845–2130		
5'8"	126–146	1890–2190		
5'9"	130–151	1950–2265		
5'10"	133–156	1995–2340		
5'11"	137–161	2055–2415		
6'0"	141–166	2115–2490		

Adapted from: U.S. Department of Agriculture, Home and Garden Bulletin No. 74.

From the chart, you can see if you are overweight. If you don't know how to count calories, I suggest you go to the nearest bookstore and buy yourself a calorie counter. Then become aware of how much it costs you (in calories) to eat that extra bite of food or piece of chocolate cake or apple pie. You might want to adapt my evaluation formula for food: I mentally weigh a dessert by asking myself, "Is it going to taste good enough to cost me 500 calories?" If it's an exceptional dessert, my answer is yes. If not, I pass it up.

But one way to be sure I don't eat that kind of stuff is to not buy it and not have it around the house. We keep very little "junk food" in the pantry. That's my form of willpower. What's yours?

Junk food is not what makes our bodies the magnificent works they are—so intricately designed that no electronic device has been able to duplicate them. Our body is the greatest gift God has given us (with the exception of eternal life through His Son) and yet we abuse, neglect, overfeed, undernourish it, and let it grow stiff. That's no way to treat our most prized possession.

Right now, would you make the commitment to no longer abuse your body?

Assignment: **Feeling Fabulous With Your Body**

1. Make a commitment to yourself to take care of your body.
2. Read and practice *The Weekend Athlete's Way to a Pain Free Monday* by Hyman Jampol.
3. After one month of stretching, enroll in a physical fitness program to get your body back to your proper weight and shape.
4. Reread the calorie chart and circle the number of calories you should have daily according to your height.
5. On the calorie chart, write in your present weight and your daily calorie intake.
6. Make an effort to eat no more than your body requires according to the chart.
7. Faithfully begin and stick with the exercises in this chapter.

*Some women grow more beautiful as they
mature.*

ARLENE DAHL

7

Beautiful You

*She makes herself coverings; her clothing is
fine linen and purple.*[1]

We have covered a lot of ground in the last few chapters—all
extremely important at forty-plus—to help you develop an
ageless attitude so you can feel fabulous in every way possible.

As you have seen, growing beautiful is a long process and
must be built from within first. Feeling fabulous on the inside,
you'll radiate a fabulous, glowing outer image as well.

Every woman wants to be beautiful. But, let's face it. Most of
us were not given a perfect set of features or a face that doesn't
require a bit of help here and there to make it more attractive.
Rebecca Hinman, a self-improvement expert and co-owner of
S.I. Seminars,* says that she doesn't know of one face that
cannot be made prettier.

In this chapter you will learn how to choose the most becoming colors so you can look fabulous at any age. You will
also learn how to evaluate and plan a wardrobe that will save

---

* Rebecca Hinman and Ann Ellis are owners of S.I. Seminars in the Portland, Oregon, area. S.I. Seminars are dedicated to self-improvement of the
whole woman on an individual basis or through seminars which are held nationwide. For more information, write: 3580 N.W. Ashland Place, Beaverton,
Oregon 97006, or phone 503-244-2694 or 503-645-8004.

you money and time, while increasing its versatility. But first, I'd like you to think about how you usually look and feel the first thing in the morning. Not too fabulous? If you are a work-at-home woman, you may not have the incentive to look fabulous as soon as you get up.

Several years ago while I was rearing my two youngsters, Tim and Tobi, and being an at-home mother and wife, I'd get up and throw on any comfortable old thing, with no regard to color coordination or style. After all, I wasn't going anyplace so why dress up? But I soon learned that often I felt the way I looked. If I looked dowdy, I felt dowdy.

That realization caused me to change my ways. It really didn't take any longer to dress with care than to look sloppy—even for staying home. The rewards were great—and still are!

I have talked with several women who feel the effects of how they look in the morning. Those who have changed from sloppy to sharp in the morning have been happier for it. Not only do they feel better, but if something comes up unexpectedly, like an invitation to lunch with their husbands, they are ready at a moment's notice.

Being well-groomed is important. Several years ago I attended a retreat and can remember well the radiant young woman who spoke on the subject of grooming. Having just become a Christian, one of the changes in her life was the importance of her physical appearance. Her old philosophy had been: "Why should I care how I look—I don't have to see myself."

But she soon realized one of the responsibilities of being a Christian was to release the old image and "put on a new face." Then she adorned herself as did the holy women who hoped in God.[2]

Some women have misunderstood the biblical interpretation of *adornment.* The original Greek translation says: "not to *only* use outward adornment." The word *only* has been left out of later translations and many women believe adornment to be sinful.[3]

Adornment is not sinful, so "if the barn needs painting, paint it," advises Charles Swindoll[4] in his *Insight for Living* tapes.*

Like anything else, adornment can be a detriment if it becomes an obsession and pushes God out of His rightful place in our lives. Moderation, cleanliness, being well-groomed with a soft feminine appearance is pleasing to look at and is an expression of love and concern for ourselves as well as those who must look at and be with us each day.

You may be thinking, "I don't need any of Ruby's advice. I keep my mind healthy, I exercise, I wear the latest fashions, have my hair done, and use makeup. I already look fabulous."

Well, that's wonderful if you do. But I find that I can always learn something more to make myself just a little bit more attractive. So, I hope you'll stick with me.

Color

I love color! Although I've always known I felt better in certain colors (like fuschia and burgundy) and uncomfortable with others (like black and pure white), I only recently learned the reasons why.

Various color experts around the country tell us that women respond naturally to certain colors. But by forty-plus, we may have lost that built-in color sense. When that happens, we buy clothing because a color happens to be "in" this season or because it looks beautiful on a friend. That is the wrong basis, however, on which to build a practical and lasting wardrobe. Of course, the clothing industry wants to sell new garments every season, so they tempt us with fresh, exciting colors.

To help you avoid impulse buying and choosing less-than-fabulous colors, I have included a *chromatic scale* that divides women into four categories. To make finding your own colors more fun, and because most women dream of owning a fur of

* Charles Swindoll is a popular author and Christian leader. His radio program, "Insight for Living," is heard on more than 100 stations.

their very own, I have given you a distinctive mink. That mink will be your color key to the fabulous world of color for clothing, makeup, and hair.

You are about to find out which mink is most becoming to you. Are you a *Dramatic Mink?* an *Exquisite Mink?* a *Sporty Mink?* or a *Romantic Mink?*

When you discover your own personal chroma (color scale), you'll not only look fabulous when you wear "your mink," you'll eliminate costly mistakes when you purchase clothing, makeup, and all the other accessories you use and wear to make you look fabulous at forty-plus.

According to Rebecca Hinman's expert advice, finding your personal chromatic scale is the first step toward creating a totally coordinated, radiant self, at forty-plus.

Right now, check the following charts for characteristics that best describe you. As you look over the lists, keep in mind whether your skin tone is pink, white, beige, or black. With a red felt pen, check off the characteristics that best describe you in each of the three categories. It will then become apparent which "mink" you are.

You'll want to make the decision very carefully, as to which mink feels best. I have determined that I wear Exquisite Mink best. My skin is pinkish-beige; I blush easily; I was born blonde, went to dishwater brown, then to frosted blonde; and my eyes are green or blue, depending on what I wear. And I feel fabulous when I wear the chromatic scale of lavenders through burgundy.

The Fabulous Colors in Clothing

Once you've determined which chromatic mink is yours, you're ready to think about the chroma for your clothing. Some mornings I go to my closet and select something that makes me feel less than fabulous. What's wrong? The color, of course. In the first three chapters we discussed how your body, mind, and soul must be in harmony. Color, too, must be in har-

DRAMATIC MINK

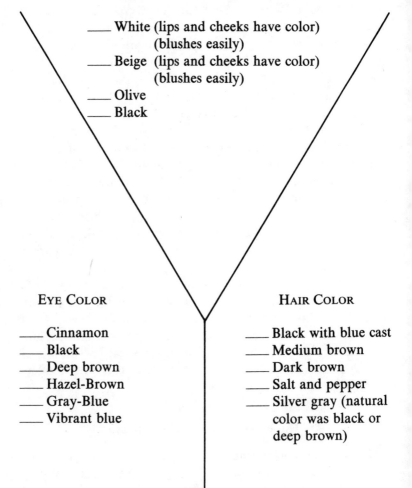

SKIN COLOR

___ White (lips and cheeks have color)
　　　(blushes easily)
___ Beige (lips and cheeks have color)
　　　(blushes easily)
___ Olive
___ Black

EYE COLOR

___ Cinnamon
___ Black
___ Deep brown
___ Hazel-Brown
___ Gray-Blue
___ Vibrant blue

HAIR COLOR

___ Black with blue cast
___ Medium brown
___ Dark brown
___ Salt and pepper
___ Silver gray (natural
　　　color was black or
　　　deep brown)

Chart courtesy of S. I. Seminars,
Portland, Oregon.

EXQUISITE MINK

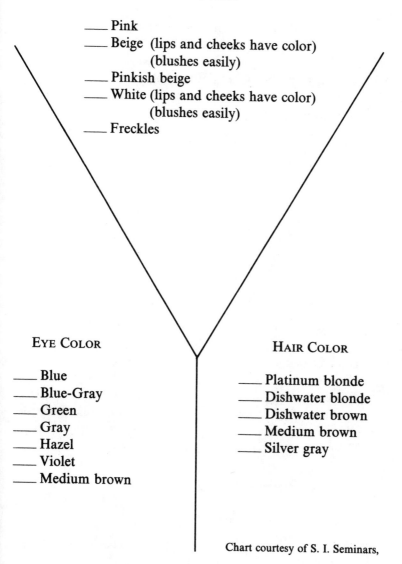

SKIN COLOR

___ Pink
___ Beige (lips and cheeks have color)
      (blushes easily)
___ Pinkish beige
___ White (lips and cheeks have color)
      (blushes easily)
___ Freckles

EYE COLOR

___ Blue
___ Blue-Gray
___ Green
___ Gray
___ Hazel
___ Violet
___ Medium brown

HAIR COLOR

___ Platinum blonde
___ Dishwater blonde
___ Dishwater brown
___ Medium brown
___ Silver gray

Chart courtesy of S. I. Seminars,

SPORTY MINK

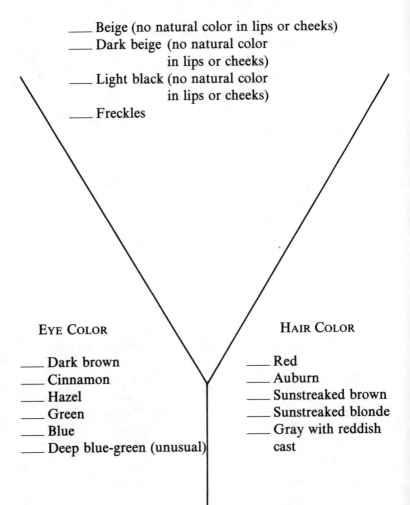

SKIN COLOR

___ Beige (no natural color in lips or cheeks)
___ Dark beige (no natural color
    in lips or cheeks)
___ Light black (no natural color
    in lips or cheeks)
___ Freckles

EYE COLOR

___ Dark brown
___ Cinnamon
___ Hazel
___ Green
___ Blue
___ Deep blue-green (unusual)

HAIR COLOR

___ Red
___ Auburn
___ Sunstreaked brown
___ Sunstreaked blonde
___ Gray with reddish
    cast

Chart courtesy of S. I. Seminars,

ROMANTIC MINK

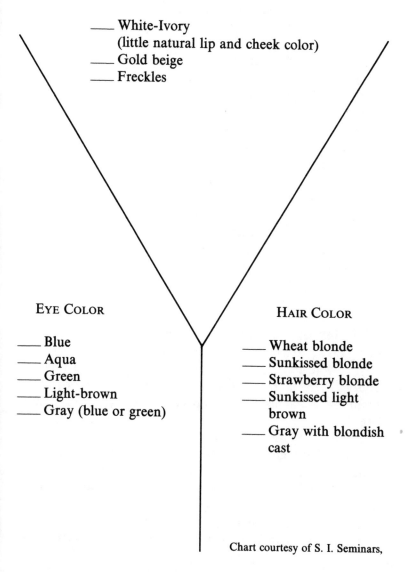

SKIN COLOR

___ White-Ivory
(little natural lip and cheek color)
___ Gold beige
___ Freckles

EYE COLOR

___ Blue
___ Aqua
___ Green
___ Light-brown
___ Gray (blue or green)

HAIR COLOR

___ Wheat blonde
___ Sunkissed blonde
___ Strawberry blonde
___ Sunkissed light
brown
___ Gray with blondish
cast

Chart courtesy of S. I. Seminars,

mony with your skin tone, your eyes, hair, the mood you're in, as well as your personality type. The colors you wear should represent you at forty-plus and feeling fabulously beautiful.

Even though you find the colors which compliment you most, remember that the intensity of color you need may change, depending on how tan or pale you are. Just the other day I was dressing for a wedding and planned to wear a wine-colored dress I'd purchased last summer. Since my skin is not as tan, the dress didn't look well on me this season. I needed more color intensity to keep me from looking washed out. Sometimes a bright scarf can add that color.

Knowing your correct color for dressing to look fabulous can also save you time when you're shopping. My friend Eileen commented, "Now when I go shopping, my eyes go straight for my own colors and I don't even bother with the rest of the stuff on the racks."

Eileen and her daughter attended a color-analysis class to learn about their chromatic scale and were given a packet of fabric in their own chroma. Eileen carries the tiny packet in her handbag and whips it out when she goes shopping. She never has to guess if the color is right or whether it will coordinate—she checks with her swatches and buys smartly! Looks smart, too!

Another way to get the color swatches is by saving a tiny two-inch square of fabric from the hems of new clothes you buy. If you are short, as I am, and must rehem everything, finding spare fabric is no problem. I staple the fabric into a small folder and have a handy packet for carrying in my handbag.

Before we think about going shopping for a new wardrobe, let's wade through the smooth, clear texture of color and learn which colors will make you look fabulous at forty-plus. You have determined which mink is for you. Now study the colors for your own chromatic scale and compare the ones you've been wearing to see how close or far off you may be.

If your colors are off, don't throw out your entire wardrobe.

Practicality is the key these days. Scarves, blouses, and makeup in the correct colors can make you feel fabulous, even though your wardrobe feels drab.

On the following pages, you'll find the chromatic scale for clothing, according to the mink you've determined is yours. As you will see, the *base colors* are practical, classic colors that will carry you from one season to the next without proclaiming the year they were purchased.

The *accent colors* are those you can be frivolous with when you have extra money to spend or want to keep your wardrobe looking fashionable according to today's trends. These can be used for accessories such as blouses, scarves, belts, costume jewelry, and whatever catches your eye as a trendy "in" item. You won't want to spend much money on these because they may only be fashionable one season.

Now, with your red felt pen, check off those colors in your personal chromatic scale. Then study them.

The Romantic-Mink and Exquisite-Mink blondes will want to be cautious about using colors that are too bright. Both their clothing and makeup should lean toward lighter colors. They must also be careful about wearing colors such as beige, which is close to the color tone of their hair. When beige is worn, it should have an accent color close to the face, so you don't fade away.

Another important tip from S. I. Seminars' Rebecca Hinman is to create only one focal point when you're dressing. For instance, an orange scarf and a pair of orange shoes keep the eyes jumping from feet to neck. The only focal point you want to create is toward your face.

Why is the *right color* so important? "It smooths and clarifies your complexion; minimizes lines, shadows, and circles; brings a healthy color to your face. Your face will pop out, pushing the color into the background."[5]

You'll also want to know how the *wrong color* can sabotage you: "Makes your complexion look pale, sallow or muddy; will accentuate lines or shadows around the mouth and nose, dark

WARDROBE CHROMATIC SCALE

Dramatic Mink

BASE COLORS (includes complete spectrum in each color)
Black
White
Forest green
Dark green
Blue-Gray
Navy
Charcoal

ACCENT COLORS
Blue (all shades including electric blue)
Green (all shades from pale green to light khaki)
Light to medium gray
Slate
Gray-Brown
Lilac
Blue-Purple (all shades)
Purple
Dusty rose
Burgundy
Cherry
Ruby red
Red-Purple

Chart courtesy of S.I. Seminars.

WARDROBE CHROMATIC SCALE

EXQUISITE MINK

BASE COLORS (includes complete spectrum of color in the lighter colors)
Royal dark blue
Navy
Light or medium dark gray
Steel Blue-Gray
Deep purple
Gray-Brown
Teal
Ash green

ACCENT COLORS
Beige
Pale gray
Lilac
Purple
Violet
Blue-Purple
Blue
Powder blue
Slate blue
Mauve
Pink
Dusty pink
Peach
Medium green
Light khaki green

Chart courtesy of S.I. Seminars.

WARDROBE CHROMATIC SCALE

SPORTY MINK

BASE COLORS (includes complete spectrum in each color)
Khaki green, light to dark
Reddish medium brown
Burnt orange, light to dark
Gray-Beige
Dark brown
Poppy

ACCENT COLORS
Mint green
Olive
Mustard
Beige
Light Gray-Beige
Cream
Winter white
Peach
Dusty rose
Pink-Peach
Burgundy

Chart courtesy of S.I. Seminars.

WARDROBE CHROMATIC SCALE

ROMANTIC MINK

BASE COLORS (includes complete spectrum of color in the lighter colors)

Cream
Camel tan
Khaki green, light to dark
Burnt orange
Russet brown

ACCENT COLORS

Cream
Ivory
Beige
Light yellow
Bright yellow
Gold
Light tones of peach
Dusty peach
Mint green
Light dull green
Olive
All greens between mint and olive

Chart courtesy of S.I. Seminars.

circles under the eyes; will accentuate blotches, if any; may age your face; will look too strong or too weak. The color tends to pop out, pushing your face into the background."[6]

You'll want to check those points when trying on clothes. As a blonde, I have to be extremely careful of not looking pale. I keep a large selection of brightly colored scarves to wear with blacks or whites that tend to phase out my face. If scarves have not been part of your wardrobe plan, let me urge you to include them. The salespeople in department stores will be more than happy to instruct you in tying them. Many have little booklets they will give you with sketches on "how-to."

Which Type Are You?

Each mink has its own distinctive personality—or does it? I know that women resent being placed into a particular category, for we are flexible, have many moods, are adaptable to our environment, and wear many different hats.

We often think of Dramatic Mink as being a dark-haired beauty who wears exotic clothes with sleek lines. But she also enjoys wearing a pair of jeans and a casual shirt. When she dresses for evening, she becomes a different person from the one who dashes to pick up groceries, or who attends a business luncheon.

Blondes, too, have been stereotyped. All too often, blondes are portrayed as sex symbols, or scatterbrained women. You may be an Exquisite Mink or Romantic Mink who enjoys wearing a sexy dress when you go to dinner. Or you may enjoy wearing ruffles upon occasion—or even a sleek, exotic dress like your sister, Dramatic Mink. But you also enjoy wearing a casual suit. There are times for jeans and shirts and sweaters.

Sporty Mink may wear vibrant colors. She may enjoy casual clothes such as a blazer and pants, but when evening comes, she may blossom out in a sleek, sexy dress that keeps the man in her life fascinated and enchanted.

Each of us has our personal signature in clothes. Sometimes

it is determined through financial circumstances. Other times it may be determined because we have been too conservative to venture out into a new look. One of the things your ageless attitude requires is that you step out—break old molds—and create a new image.

Finding a new personality in clothing can be fun! It's part of the excitement of being forty-plus and looking fabulous. For more information on wardrobe selection, read Joanne Wallace's forthcoming book *Dress With Style*.

Shoes and Handbags

Even for shoes, there is a basic rule: "They should be the same color as the hem of the garment or darker."[7] For a well-coordinated wardrobe, two wisely chosen pairs of shoes will suffice.

For handbags, one in a neutral color to blend with your outfit for daytime—and one for evening—are all you need.

A Basic Wardrobe

Earlier I said I'd suggest a basic wardrobe for you to think about. From the colors you selected from your chromatic scale of minks, chart out a coordinated wardrobe on the form that follows. The colors should blend so well that you can mix and match and make several different outfits from the basics. Copy this form on another piece of paper and work with your colors until you devise a plan with which you are happy. You'll want to coordinate around some of the items already in your closet, if they are colors that make you look and feel fabulous.

After you have completed on paper the color coordination of your basic wardrobe, study it for several days. Be sure you have come up with a harmonious color plan—one that will mix and match. The ultimate criterion is how well each item of clothing looks on you and whether you feel fabulous while you are wearing it.

Item of clothing	Cold-weather Wardrobe	Warm-weather Wardrobe
Blazer or jacket		
Skirt		
Pants		
Casual pants		
Casual skirt		
Blouse (tailored)		
Blouse (casual)		
Blouse (dressy)		
Sweater (pullover)		
Sweater (cardigan)		
Party pants		
Party blouse		
Dress (shirtwaist)		
Dress (for evening)		
Basic coat (solid color)		
Rain coat (solid color)		
Dressy shoes		
Casual shoes		
Handbag (day)		
Handbag (evening)		
Scarves		
Jewelry		

As I conclude this section on clothing, here's one last suggestion for controlling your wardrobe. It's one I use and have taught my daughters to use with success. When August rolls around and thoughts turn to buying school clothes, I ask the girls to make a chart of all the clothing they can still wear, along with the colors.

Then, at the bottom of the page, they write in what they need to buy that will coordinate with what they already have. That way, they'll have a planned, coordinated wardrobe, instead of buying whatever appeals to them "because it's so-o-o cute, Mom."

I use the same method for myself twice a year—in the spring, when thoughts turn to fun in the sun and again in the fall, when cold weather begins to tease. Although I love sunshine, the Pacific Northwest's mild winter is my favorite season for dressing; wool pants, sweaters, and blazers are my favorites.

Most of my buying is done during sales—I rarely pay full price. I have found that by anticipating my needs in advance, I seldom have to rush out to buy something for a special occasion.

For purposes of inventory and planning, I use a large piece of bookkeeping paper, but a regular sheet of paper will do nicely. Study the following form, then design a similar one, adapting it to your own needs.

First, across the top of the paper, I code the fabrics that my wardrobe consists of so I won't have to keep writing them out.

After I record the inventory of clothes on hand, I carefully decide what I need for the season to keep my wardrobe fresh and fashionable. I write those items at the bottom of the section in red ink, indicating the color I plan to buy. In the fall and spring when the fashion catalogs arrive from my favorite department stores, I check them over for two reasons: one, to see what is happening in the fashion world; and the other, to see what will fit into my *planned wardrobe*. It's also a good time to comparison-price shop with minimum effort.

As an example, if I had a brown blazer, camel wool pants, a

CLOTHING INVENTORY PLANNER

P = polyester	W = wool	V = velvet
RS = raw silk	C = corduroy	SW = suede
S = silk	CT = cotton	L = leather

Blazers	Pants	Blouses	Sweaters	Skirts	Dresses	Shoes	Scarves
SW Rose	W Burg.	S Gray Burg.	W Wine	W Gray		SW Gray.	S Rose Gray

camel wool skirt, and an oatmeal sweater, I might want to buy a brown-camel-oatmeal striped blouse to tie it all together. So I would write that at the bottom of the blouse column, in red ink. Then I could see at a glance what I would purchase.

Wardrobe planning can be fun—if you look for clothes to make you look fabulous at forty-plus!

Assignment: **Beautiful You**

1. From your own distinctive mink, choose the chromatic scale that will become your personal signature.
2. List the colors that you know make you feel fabulous:

3. Think about the type of clothing that appeals to you. If someone gave you $1,000 to spend on clothing, what would you buy?

4. Complete filling in the colors for your basic wardrobe. Study department-store displays or magazines for additional ideas.
5. Inventory your wardrobe systematically. Use the suggested form and method. Study your own wardrobe to see how you can improve upon what you already have, keeping in mind appropriate color and life-style.

Art quickens nature; Care will make a face;
Neglected beauty perisheth apace.

ROBERT HERRICK

8

It's Fun to Make Up

... A desire fulfilled is a tree of life.[1]

In the last chapter you learned that color makes a difference in how you feel and how you look. Even though your chromatic scale can help you feel fabulous in your clothes, there's still more to learn. Using the correct chroma for your makeup can make you look even more fabulous at forty-plus. However, for that fabulous look, your makeup must not be alien to your natural skin tone.

How many times have you wasted money on oh-so-pretty lipstick, that was not so on your lips. Knowing your chroma is the way to eliminate costly, ghastly errors.

Contrary to the cosmetic commercials and ads we see daily, we do not need a different set of makeup to match our clothing—IF—our clothing harmonizes and is within "our" chromatic scale. One set of makeup should blend with our entire wardrobe.

Every woman who is forty-plus and wants to look and feel fabulous must develop good color and fashion sense. There are few women of any age who can use all the makeup advertised and not look like a cosmetic commercial. Ads are purposely overemphasized to sell products. It's up to your good sense to glean what will enhance your particular type of beauty.

Because good cosmetics cost a lot, I don't recommend the trial-and-error method. Take advantage of the free makeup consultations offered at most major department stores. There is no obligation to buy.

Having a makeup demonstration can help you keep up with the trends. Makeup applied a la sixties or early seventies can date you as fast as outmoded clothing. Take Rhoda for instance. She and her husband run a charter boat off the coast of Mexico. They are both forty-plus with active ageless attitudes.

Rhoda's tiny figure is perfect for the western fashions she loves. From behind, Rhoda's thick brown hair helps to form the ageless image. But when she turns, you are greeted with heavy, tar-painted, half-moon eyebrows and blood-red lips that overstate their natural contour.

The incorrect application and colors of makeup have ruined Rhoda's image. Although she is a lovely, gentle, sensitive woman, with a delightful sense of humor, her makeup paints a very different picture.

Harsh, outmoded makeup can ruin your image, too. Makeup should have no other purpose than to make you more attractive, in a natural, pleasing way. Keeping within your chromatic scale will help eliminate that unnatural look.

Foundation

"When choosing your foundation, it is always wise to remember that makeup should *enhance* your beauty, not mask your face," says Portland, Oregon's Young Career Woman of the Year and first runner-up in the Mrs. (Oregon) America competition, Rebecca Hinman.

Makeup should be so natural that only *you* know you're wearing it. There should be no telltale chin line to give your beauty secrets away.

There's really no secret to selecting the correct foundation— once you understand your skin color. The best way to do that is to make a test run! Rebecca advises her students to go into a department store and test wear a sample of the foundation they choose, *before* they buy it. See how that color looks on you in the sunlight, in the car, and in your office or home. Live with it a day. Then decide if the color is right for you.

Don't let a salesperson make that decision for you. Many are not properly trained. Their lack of experience can be costly to you, besides creating a less than fabulous image at forty-plus.

It all sounds so confusing, doesn't it? It really isn't if you begin by looking at your face. If you have natural color in your lips and cheeks, you'll need an ivory underbase.

If you have little or no color in your lips and cheeks, your underbase should have a hint of pink.

Most models use makeup sponges to apply foundation smoothly and evenly, says Rebecca, who has modeled extensively in Spain and whose fashion-magazine credits include *Glamour* and *Vogue*.

Following is the chromatic scale that will give your skin a fabulous glow at forty-plus.

Foundation Color Tones

Dramatic Mink: Ivory, beige or brown (possibly with slight pink undertone)

Exquisite Mink: Ivory or beige (possibly with slight pink undertone)

Sporty Mink: Brown or beige (peach tone or slightly pinkish)

Romantic Mink: Warm peach tones or slightly pinkish cast

Blush and Lip Color

Choosing the right color foundation blends all the different skin tones of your face together for a smooth, pleasing-to-the-eye effect. So remember, when you choose your blush and lip

BLUSH AND LIP COLOR

MINK	BLUSH SHADES	LIP COLOR
DRAMATIC MINK	Ruby red (avoid red with orange tones Rose Pinks Burgundy Mauve	Plum pink Ruby Red Burgundy
EXQUISITE MINK	Rose Blue-Pink Burgundy	Pastels Plum Mauve Burgundy
SPORTY MINK	Orange Ginger Peach (avoid pink tones) Rust	Rust Brick Coral Peach Orange
ROMANTIC MINK	Peach Coral	Warm deep pink Coral Peach

Chart courtesy of S. I. Seminars.

color, it should never resemble an SOS from your face. You want your lips and cheeks to look like a natural part of you, rather than draw attention to themselves.

Because you don't want to flash like a beacon, you'll want to be sure the intensity of color is right also. Your age, the amount of color you already have in your lips and cheeks, how dark or fair your skin is, and the color and style of your clothes will all play a part in determining the right shades of lip color and blush for you.

Carefully look over and study the guide on the previous page to find the correct shades to make you look and feel fabulous.

Eye Makeup

Cruising along at a gentle speed, let's move on from lips and cheeks, and point upward to your eyes—those lovely pools of color that are often referred to as the windows of your soul.

This morning my husband and our youngsters were having breakfast in a small cafe not far from our boat moorage. The waitress was outstanding—not for her service—but for the color of her metallic-blue eyelids!

Apparently, she never learned that the object of wearing eye shadow is to enhance the shape and color of eyes—not to let everyone know she has them.

The rule for eyes is the same as for the rest of your face. Natural—subtle—blend—natural—natural—natural!

You'll be able to enhance the shape and color of your fabulous eyes by finding your chroma, then choosing the appropriate color according to your own eye color on the following charts. The colors are recommended for eyelids. Use a lighter shade of the same color, or ivory, for highlighter under brows.

Selecting the correct color for your eyes is only the first step toward becoming more fabulous to look at. Proper application is as important. Department-store makeup consultants (not salespeople), who represent various cosmetic companies, will make you up by appointment, at no charge. Also, there are nu-

EYE SHADOW

DRAMATIC MINK

BROWN-BLACK EYE COLOR

> Cream
> Gray-Brown
> Gray
> Navy
> Smoky navy
> Deep blue
> Hunter green
> Burgundy
> Purple
> Raspberry
> Smoky plum

BLUE-GRAY EYE COLOR

> Cream
> Gray
> Dark blue
> Ash blue
> Blue-Black
> Ash purple

Chart courtesy of S. I. Seminars.

EYE SHADOW

EXQUISITE MINK

LIGHT BROWN-GRAY EYE COLOR

Cream
Gray
Gray-Brown
Red-Brown
Rose
Violet
Mauve
Plum

GREEN EYE COLOR

Cream
Gray
Ash gray
Deep smoky green
Ash green

BLUE / BLUE-GRAY
EYE COLOR

Cream
Beige
Gray
Smoky blue
Navy
Plum
Mauve

Chart courtesy of S. I. Seminars.

EYE SHADOW

SPORTY MINK

BROWN EYE COLOR

Beige
Brown
Medium brown
Rust
Cinnamon
Apricot
Peach
Charcoal
Gray-Brown

AMBER EYE COLOR

Beige
Brown
Light brown
Medium brown
Gray-Brown
Charcoal
Rust
Apricot
Peach

GREEN EYE COLOR

Beige
Brown
Medium brown
Dark brown
Khaki
Deep green
Muted green
Charcoal
Gray-Brown
Apricot

Chart courtesy of S. I. Seminars.

EYE SHADOW

ROMANTIC MINK

LIGHT BROWN-GRAY EYE COLOR

Cream
Ivory
Beige
Light brown
Dark brown
Charcoal
Cinnamon
Rust
Peach

BLUE-GRAY EYE COLOR

Cream
Ivory
Light brown
Dark brown
Gray-Brown
Charcoal
Deep green
Deep blue
Navy
Smoky turquoise

GREEN EYE COLOR

Cream
Ivory
Beige
Brown
Gray-Brown
Khaki
Deep green
Smoky medium green

Chart courtesy of S. I. Seminars.

merous salons across the country that specialize in proper makeup application.

Rebecca applies her modeling and beauty expertise through S. I. Seminars, where you get individual, personal makeup application. Many other salons across the nation offer this same service.

What Am I Buying?

As you browse the cosmetic counters and begin reading labels of the products you use, you may wonder about what those enormously long words mean and how pure the item is. Rebecca has taken the mystery away with the list below. But first, she advises us that all cosmetics sold in the United States must have preservatives added. The most common are: *methylparaben* and *propylparaben,* so don't be misled by paying higher prices for items that claim to be natural or organic.

You can save money by comparing ingredients. Why pay twelve dollars or more for a cosmetic that has the very same ingredients as a five-dollar item? You may want to copy the following list of ingredients onto a small piece of paper you can keep in your handbag for easy reference so you know what you are buying.

Most common ingredients found in cosmetics:

Water: base
Mineral oil: emollient (softens or soothes)
Glycerol monodistearate: emulsifier (bonder of agents)
Synthetic spermaceti: waxy, emollient, protector
Glycerin: emollient, humectant
Stearic acid: texturizer, adds lustre
Peg 8 stearate: emulsifier
Cetyl alcohol: waxy emollient, protector
Triethanolamine: emulsifier
Methylparaben: preservative
Propylparaben: preservative

Vitamin E: antioxidant, preservative, healer
Vitamin C: antioxidant, preservative
Ascorbyl palmitate: antioxidant, preservative
Peg 12:   emollient, emulsifier
Amphoteric 6:   cleanser
Lipal 300 W: emulsifier, cleanser
Propylene glycol: solvent or tonic
Lanolin fraction: conditioner
Imidazolidinyl urea: preservative
Sodium borate: emulsifier, antiseptic, astringent
Polysorbate 20:   emulsifier
Quaternium 15:   antiseptic
Fragrance: odor
FD & C Red: color

Glasses

Not only do styles in eye makeup change, but in glasses as well. The woman with an ageless attitude who is creating a new outer image won't want to spoil the total look by wearing frames that look as though they were custom designed for a Siamese cat. Improper frames can distort your whole face if the shape and color are wrong.

At forty-plus, many women are wearing glasses, but still think of them as a domestic necessity rather than a fashion item. When you consider that glasses are worn every day and are the first thing people see on your face, you wonder why women don't treat them as a number-one beauty accessory.

When choosing frames, never make the decision while your eyes are still dilated after an exam. Look over the frames and think about them before ordering.

Some of the things you'll want to consider are: the shape of your face; the color of your hair; your hairstyle.

If you have a square face, frames with a softer line such as oval or round may look best on you. For a full, round face, try a frame with a different shape.

The important thing is not to overpower your face with frames that are too heavy looking, either in shape or color. The Exquisite Minks and Romantic Minks will want softly colored frames to enhance their hair and complexion. But by contrast, Dramatic Mink and Sporty Mink will choose darker frames.

Color and fashion can be fun and challenging. Recently my close friend Sally became aware of color. Although an attractive woman not yet forty-plus, color consciousness actually rejuvenated her. It was fun watching Sally blossom out in a colorful wardrobe and a lively face. She even had her copious strawberry blonde hair cut into a chic style worthy of a woman who wants to feel fabulous.

Change can be yours merely for the deciding. Completing the following assignment will help you make change a bit easier to accomplish.

Assignment: **It's Fun to Make Up**

1. In this chapter, reread the section on foundation. Check off the color best suited to your unique characteristics. Now check it against the foundation you are already wearing to find out if you need to change color.
2. Start a list. Make a note of the correct foundation color.
3. In the section Blush and Lip Color, check off the colors most flattering to your skin tone. Be sure they blend with your wardrobe. Jot the color tones on your list.
4. Study the charts on eyeshadow and check off the colors that are right for you. Add those to your list.
5. Before buying any of the items on your list, ask for a free consultation at a major department store. Watch the expert as she applies your makeup. Talk over the colors you have picked out from the color charts; ask her to use those colors on you.
6. Check over your glasses to see if they're fashionable, flattering, and make you look fabulous. If not, as soon as you can afford to, have your frames changed.

Where in the world are you going (with your hair up in curlers) that is more important than where you are right now?

AUTHOR UNKNOWN

9

Your Crowning Glory

*Even the hairs of your head are numbered.
. . . you are of more value than many sparrows*[1]

There's one more important item we must cover before we leave the matter of changing your outer image to that becoming to a woman who is Forty-Plus and Feeling Fabulous. Your hair! Mothers have always told their daughters: "Your hair is your crowning glory." But some women must not believe it.

Women who neglect their hair or wear unflattering styles are telling the world just that. Those unflattering hairstyles we see so many of tell us how much we need our hair to make us look more attractive. There are few women who could manage to have their heads shaved and still look fabulous at forty-plus or any other age. Hair is an important part of the outer image by which people form their first snap-decision impression of us. If a woman's hair is clean, styled, and flattering, the impression she makes is decidedly different from that of an unkempt, oily mess. Your hair is the frame for your face.

Style and Cut

Unfortunately, by the time many women reach forty-plus, their frame has become a "menopause bob." And with it, has gone most of the crowning glory and femininity that an ageless face needs for softness in order to look and feel fabulous.

What is this phenomenon that happens to women as they near the middle years? I'm not sure. There seems to be an unwritten rule that is secretly transmitted to every woman over thirty-five: "You should never wear long hair again—it must be short, neat and controlled."

But, "nothing could be farther from the truth. The proof is that the world's most glamorous ageless women, with a few exceptions, prefer longer hairstyles. Their hair is voluminous, luxuriant, a veritable mane . . . they all have a quality of elegant disarray." Touchable hair is one of our most feminine physical qualities. Hair is sexy.[2] Female country-western singers have always known this. No menopause bobs for them!

I'm not talking about hair that reaches past your shoulders. That can be as aging as the menopause bob. If you prefer to wear your hair longer, it should be swept off your face. Gravity tends to pull the face down; that's why we need to keep our hair on the "up" side.

Long hair or longish hair should have some kind of movement—layering, soft curls, waves. Some of the outstanding forty-plus-and-looking-fabulous women, like Princess Grace and Jacqueline Kennedy Onassis, still have fullness and movement in their hairstyles.

Another consideration in finding the right style to look fabulous at forty-plus is the shape of your face. It's essential to consider whether your face is square, round, diamond shaped, or pear-shaped. Some women are lucky enough to have a perfect oval. But if your face is other than an oval, select a hairstyle in which the fullness of your hair softens angular corners, too-strong jaws, receding chins, or low foreheads, advises Joanne Wallace in her book *The Image of Loveliness.*[3]

Many women use a center part, but it can be hazardous to your beauty since it cuts facial features in half, rather than creating an overall look that flows together. It also forces you to try to style both sides of your hair exactly the same. That is virtually impossible because of the natural way hair grows. My own hairdresser, Kathleen Harlan, cautions that since no one has a perfectly symmetrical face, a center part only accentuates those differences.

Kathleen, though not yet forty-plus, is well on her way to developing an ageless attitude, so she will be looking and feeling as fabulous then as she does now.

As styles director for *Hair With Interest* shops in Milwaukie, Oregon, looking fabulous is Kathleen's business, and she knows that arriving at the proper cut is perhaps more important than style. She believes that a precision cut is what enables a woman to achieve a style without effort. Just what is a precision cut? It is when the stylist works with the unique growth pattern of your hair while she is cutting it.

If hair is cut properly, it should just fall into place nicely. But when hair has been cut improperly, you have hassles, because you are trying to work against the natural growth pattern. It makes me think of trying to iron out a porcupine—an impossible task!

Besides being a battle of the hairs, the wrong style can also create an immediate impression of inflexibility, repression, or sexlessness—none of which is part of the ageless-attitude agenda.

When selecting a style, remember that many things must be considered, such as your hair's texture, location of cowlicks, and even the direction of hair growth. If you have communicated with your stylist (a must!), she'll know the feeling or look you want and will do everything she can to find a happy solution for you.

Do be realistic about your request. If you have thin hair, you aren't going to get a beautiful, long, windblown look. So don't expect miracles!

Another thing to consider is your life-style. If you swim or are physically active, you might want a shorter cut that is flattering but easy to blow dry. Many women with longer hair no longer swim because hair care is too time consuming. If your style is restraining your physical activities, it's defeating its purpose in your life.

If you're in doubt about the cut that will help you look and feel more fabulous now that you're forty-plus, look at the magazines and notebooks full of hairstyles at a beauty shop. You can browse through at your leisure. Just take time to go in before you make an appointment. You might even take advantage of that time to talk with, and watch, the stylist who will be working with you. Watching her will give you a clue about the quality of work to expect.

One more thing to remember—many hair stylists do not have an ageless attitude. They may not think being forty-plus is fabulous at all, and they may try to talk you into a menopause bob. Go with determination and caution. Don't allow anyone to deter you from a new ageless hairstyle once you've decided to let go of the old look.

Hair Care and Health

Cut and style are important, but without healthy hair, no style can do you justice. Your hair is another reason to maintain good physical health.

Healthy hair reflects a healthy body—it's that simple. Pregnancy, hormones, anesthesia, and surgery all have their effect on the condition of your hair. If you've had surgery within six months to a year, a permanent may not take properly.

It's always wise to tell your hairdresser about the condition of your health and any medication you may be taking, before having color applied or a perm.

Illness, medication, and poor nutrition can affect your hair's growth, texture, thickness, and sheen. Sunlight, heated and air-conditioned rooms, extreme cold weather, chlorinated water in swimming pools, all dry your hair, as do blow dryers.

To counteract all these drying influences, conditioning is a must. Some hairdressers suggest having three different good-quality shampoos and conditioners in your bathroom. Each time you wash your hair, use a different product so your hair won't become resistant to the beneficial effects of any one.

To Dye or Not to Dye

And now, on to the fascinating world of color again. To dye or not to dye is the question many women ask at forty-plus, when we find more silver threads among the gold than not. But today, no one need be gray, except by choice.

One alternative to gray is frosting (sometimes referred to as aluminizing or foil wrap). Softly, a frost blends in natural gray with blonde. Since natural-color hair always has many highlights of different colors, a frosting leaves the same effect.

But stay away from harsh tinting and dying, warns Kathleen Harlan. It looks dated, colored, and unnatural. A tint will scream out, "Hey, everybody—I've covered my gray!" By contrast a frost gently blends the gray all together, subtly.

There are two ways to have your hair frosted. One is painful. The other is a pleasure. I have experienced both and prefer the foil-weaving method.

The old-fashioned, painful way is done with a tight rubber covering that fits your head like a bathing-cap and has several tiny holes. The hair is pulled through the holes with something like a crochet hook, just a few strands at a time. It's hurtful and time-consuming if you have longer hair. I've sat for hours while the tears rolled down my cheeks, promising myself I'd never subject myself to that torture again. It was truly a blessing when I moved to another town, and a new hairdresser suggested the foil-weaving method.

Weaving is a relatively new method of color application. (It can also be used for a reverse frost—light to dark.) Your hair is woven, creating indistinct sections. The sections that are colored become blended, eliminating streaks or stripes. An overall color change is created without all of your hair being colored. Advantage? One is that when the "grow out" becomes obvious, it can be touched up easily.

Kathleen encourages this method of frosting at forty-plus because it is excellent for "salt and pepper" hair, especially at the "mousy" stage. By weaving in one or more shades, you have a warm, shiny color and still utilize your own natural highlights.

Unfortunately, most of us are not lucky enough to gray gracefully. Once there, gray may be lovely and make you feel fabulous—but surely there's nothing wrong in helping it along in the meantime.

Kathleen agrees that not all gray needs to be frosted. If gray means "old lady" to you, then by all means color it! But if you can see yourself carrying off gray with distinction and flair, maybe you should give it a try. With the right cut, it can be quite flattering.

As your hair grays, remember that it tends to become a tad ornery, a bit more curly, and somewhat harder to manage— which scores another point for a good cut.

Choosing the Color

Not everyone can be a frosted blonde at forty-plus, so choosing the proper hair color is as important as selecting your colorful wardrobe. Many of the color experts I have talked with believe that finding a hair color that enhances your total image should be a simple matter, once you know your skin color. Hair color must liven your skin tone, rather than deaden it.

If you'll slip back into your beautiful mink for a moment, we'll see what the chromatic scale (again, courtesy of S. I. Seminars) reveals for your particular type.

Dramatic Mink: Women who fall into this category usually have color in their cheeks and lips, and their eyes are deep brown, black, or cinnamon. Because their hair is usually very dark, they should not attempt to become blondes or be tempted to frost. They should also avoid red tones. Dramatic Minks usually gray beautifully and can wear "salt and pepper" with flair, especially if the haircut is very fashionable.

Exquisite Mink: We usually have a lot of natural pink color in our cheeks and lips. Our eyes are blue, green, hazel, or gray, and our hair is light brown with a grayish cast. We can frost our hair and look very natural since we were born blonde. The ash tones are best for us. I have been graying since I was thirty and have a frame of white around my face. I enjoy being a blonde because it feels natural for me.

Sporty Mink: If you fall into this category, you probably have no color in your lips or cheeks. Your eyes are dark brown to black, or deep hazel or cinnamon, and your hair has red undertones. Usually, the graying process is not becoming to you, and you can frost if you use reddish tones. Once you've turned completely gray, however, the color may look fabulous on you if you feel comfortable with it.

Romantic Mink: Like her sporty sister, Romantic Mink also has little color in her lips and cheeks. Her eyes are usually gray, blue, green, or violet, with lovely strawberry-blonde, light-brown, or blonde hair. You, too, can look fabulous with gray hair once it has all arrived, but you may want to cover it with reddish or golden undertones in the meantime.

No matter which mink you wear, you'll want to be absolutely sure that your hair creates the most flattering frame available to you and ties in with the total concept you're trying to achieve.

Kathleen Harlan reminds the women who come to her for beauty advice that it's as important to keep their hairstyle up to date as their clothes and makeup. Nothing can make you look more unbalanced than wearing a trendy new fashion and having a 1940s hairstyle. Being forty-plus can be fun when you have a total plan for yourself, put it into effect, then emerge feeling really fabulous!

Assignment: **Your Crowning Glory**

1. Do you have gray hair?
2. Does it make you feel old?
3. Make an honest evaluation of how "gray" looks on you.
4. Decide if you want to change hair color.
5. Look through magazines to find a style that seems right for you.
6. Do you have a hairdresser you trust and have confidence in? If not, next time you see someone with a good cut, stop that person to ask the name of her hairdresser.
7. Take positive action to change those things that keep you from being forty-plus—looking and feeling fabulous. List your plan of action below in the order of priority.

   a.

   b.

   c.

   d.

   e.

Part IV

Achieving a Fabulous Marriage

*Matrimony—the high seas for which no
compass has been invented.*

HEINRICH HEINE

10

Communication: Why, How, and When

*It is not good that . . . man should be alone;
I will make . . . a helper fit for him.*[1]

Developing an ageless attitude at forty-plus and learning how to look and feel fabulous is one important part of the whole we're working toward. Another important part of that whole is marriage. The contribution a happy marriage makes to most of our lives is vital.

At forty-plus, when all too many marriages are falling apart, you'll want to evaluate where your relationship stands and insure that the foundation of your marriage stays firm and holds tough.

Ideally, these are the years that life "should" be relaxed. With the nest now empty, there should be a hint of spring fever stirring in your marriage. Thoughts of romance and a new life with your mate can now be more than a vision.

Yes, *ideally,* every marriage *should* be reenergized at forty-plus. Yet, if we're going to be realistic, we have to admit that revitalized marriages happen less and less at forty-plus. For in place of balmy Hawaiian breezes and stirring romance, many experience a Florida hurricane.

That's what happened to me. As I hit the forty-year mark, my twenty-year marriage crumbled in disaster; I experienced a bitter, heartbreaking divorce. But that painful dissolvement further expanded my ageless attitude. One of the best things to come out of that period was my determination to have a successful second marriage. That required a lot of soul-searching to find my weaknesses. I'll be sharing what I learned, in this chapter and the next few.

One of the many things I learned is how to build a firm foundation for my marriage. The Bible warns that a house built upon a rock will withstand the rains and winds, but one built on sand will fall.[2] In the next few chapters I'll be talking about the concrete that binds a husband and wife together through those intermittent winter storms.

Commitment

Today, *commitment* is a word many young people hesitate using. That is one reason why "living together" is not too satisfactory, as couples soon find out. Just recently, a twenty-four-year-old woman told me of her "divorce" from her live-in partner. She sadly reflected, "When you just live together, there is no commitment. All the little things you can't stand about each other just pile up. You know that the day will come when you won't be able to take it any longer, and you'll walk out."

The lack of commitment makes it easier to be slack on tolerance and many other things that make a satisfying relationship. Perhaps we need to define commitment. Webster says it's "an agreement or pledge to do something in the future."[3]

Most of us who are forty-plus entered our first marriages with total commitment. We pledged to put all we had into our marriages. Unfortunately, many of us did not know that "all we had" was not enough.

Anyone can be married. Not everyone has acquired the ability, the endurance, or the hope for their future to commit themselves with the kind of love that Jesus talked about in my favorite chapter of the Bible, 1 Corinthians 13. That top-quality love includes patience, kindness, and understanding.

Another key point in understanding what commitment means is to have a clear-cut definition of leadership in marriage. Today we hear much about women of all ages developing inner strength, being assertive, and becoming liberated. Each is a completely different topic, and our interest on these pages is solely in where leadership in the home is concerned.

We must not confuse inner strength with dominance. God commands: "Wives, be subject to your husbands.... for the husband is head of the wife as Christ is head of the church...."[4] These verses are getting a lot of attention, and it is important that each woman understand what the words mean and practice them, if her marriage is to be strong.

These verses do not mean that wives are to be slaves or servants to their husbands, as the word *subject* might imply to you. On the contrary, when the wife loves her husband as *she* would like to be loved, and the husband loves his wife as *he* would like to be loved, and they *both love Christ* as He loves the Church, you have a perfect circle of love. No one is servant. No one is master.

However, remember this. There must be a leader in every organization or there is chaos. And that leader is your husband. Unity and teamwork, though, is the name of the marriage game.

In my first marriage, that simple basic rule was missing. I did not understand the concept of leadership. In my second marriage, I wouldn't be without it. This is the way Tom and I employ Christ's command. First, we discuss issues. Together we try to arrive at a meeting of the minds. Then Tom sets policy and I help enforce or carry it out. We work as a team—not as master and slave.

Where children are still in the home (as in ours), this unity keeps the family strong and pulling in the same direction. Children know they can't play their games of running from one parent to another to win out, because the rules are the same at both ends. That's unity and strength. Teamwork builds a concrete foundation and is one part of your commitment to your marriage—and one that contributes to feeling fabulous.

Right now, let's take a short inventory of your marriage.

1. Check those words which best describe your marriage:

   a. Joyful   f. Tolerable
   b. Loving   g. Miserable
   c. Happy   h. Frustrating
   d. Fun   i. Boring
   e. Compatible   j. Existing
                   k. Hanging by a thread

2. Examine your commitment to your marriage. Do you have the determination to remain married?
3. If you answered no, what have been the reasons for staying in your marriage?
4. Does your marriage have a leader? Is it your husband? Do you work as a team?

The Art of Communication

It's great to know who your leader is, but there must also be communication for that leader to be effective. One of the most important elements of a marriage relationship is *conversation*. Doesn't it make you feel good and a bit envious to see a couple locked in each other's gaze, speaking softly over dinner in a quiet corner of a restaurant?

No one else is present in their world—just two people who are fascinated, interested, and obviously enjoying each other. There's no exchange of rejection, criticism, or putting down; total acceptance is their theme song. Both are on their best behavior—perhaps some sincere compliments, a bit of encouragement, smiles, some laughter, all the while holding hands.

Both are well-groomed for the occasion. Everything about them says: WE CARE ABOUT EACH OTHER.

But, "What's a couple to talk about who have been married for eternity and see each other every day of their lives?" you ask. Here's how one couple solved the problem. An elderly couple, married many years, dined out regularly at the same tiny coffee shop. Their waitress, impressed by their obvious enjoyment of each other but baffled by their endless chatter, one day inquired: "What in the world do you two find to talk about all the time?"

With a gleeful chuckle, the couple replied: "Well, we don't always have a lot to talk about. But when we run out of conversation, we take turns counting out loud from one to ten. We usually start laughing—and that brings conversation."

That elderly couple demonstrates that you must work to make conversation. Motivation also plays an important part in developing communication. One of my favorite authors is John Powell, whose tender understanding and love for people make his books very special to read. In his book *The Secret of Staying in Love,* John Powell says, "The only motive from which true dialogue can result is the desire for communication. We have said that communication means sharing and that a person shares his real self when he shares his feelings. Consequently, the only valid motive for dialogue is this desire to give to another the most precious thing I can give: myself in self-disclosure, in the transparency achieved in dialogue."[5]

Since true communication does involve risk (of exposing our innermost feelings), perhaps this is the key to why few husbands and wives are able to move into active dialogue.

Not only does communication involve risk, it also requires trust. The subconscious questions being asked are: Can I trust you? How far can I trust you? Will you understand or will you reject my feelings? Would you laugh at me or pity me?[6]

In a marriage relationship, those questions have been answered. If the answers are mostly, "No," then the dialogue will be very guarded, and the relationship will suffer because the necessary trust is not there.

To illustrate, let's take the example of a young, eager bride who was used to sharing her feelings and dreams. Every time she talked about deep needs and career plans, her new husband became critical. It didn't take long to realize that it wasn't safe to share on that level. Early in this marriage, the walls preventing dialogue were being built.

Being an extremely sensitive young woman, she just pulled her head into her shell, the same way a turtle does, and came out only when she knew it was safe.

However, had she gone a step further and explained her hurt and feelings of rejection to her new husband, he may have allowed his lovely bride to enter into his own life experience. Then real communication would be a reality to both.

Not only is trust involved in meaningful dialogue, but an interpretation of words is required. Two people can say the same words, but have a different feeling and reason for saying them. Tone of voice, eye and facial expressions, and body positions are all keys in translating and listening to the words your mate is saying to you.

But all too often, only the sounds hit our ears, and Dr. Paul Tournier, the Swiss psychiatrist and author, says, "Listen to all the conversations of our world, between nations as well as those between couples. They are for the most part, dialogues of the deaf."

And so it is with the conversations that most husbands and wives experience. It is not only sad, it is pathetic and tragic that we have not mastered the art of communication with the one person who is most important in our life—our mate.

I am going to describe five different levels of conversation that John Powell defines in more detail, in his book *Why Am I Afraid to Tell You Who I Am?* Read them carefully. Then check off those that best describe the typical communication going on between your mate and you.

Level 5: *Cliché conversation*
> This represents the weakest response and is the lowest level of self-communication. It goes: "How are you? . . . How is your family? Where have you been? I like your dress very much." The self is never exposed.

Level 4: *Reporting the facts about others*
> We expose almost nothing about ourselves—we tell what so-and-so has said or done. We give nothing of ourselves and expect nothing in return.

Level 3: *My ideas and judgments*
> Some communication of my person. I will risk telling you some of my ideas, judgments, and decisions. I am testing you with my ideas to see if you accept me.

Level 2: *My feelings (emotions) at "gut level"*
> I express the *feelings* that lie under my ideas, judgments, and convictions.

Level 1: *Peak communication*
> All deep and authentic friendships and especially the union of those who are married must be based on absolute openness and honesty.[7]

The last few pages of John Powell's book *The Secret of Staying in Love* are filled with some great conversation starters. They are meant to stimulate feelings and the communication of those feelings. I will include only a few, but suggest you use this fine book as a guide to developing the art of communication with your mate. When you ask your mate these questions, pay attention to the feelings he may not be able to express and try to help him verbalize them. Have him do the same for you.

How do I feel when—

1. You surprise me with something nice?
2. You seem to appreciate me?
3. You laugh at my jokes?
4. I think that you are not recognizing my needs?

   5. I make a mistake and you point it out?
   6. You are holding me in your arms?
   7. You seem to be rejecting my feelings?
   8. I think that you are judging me?
   9. You become violently angry with me?
 10. Others notice our closeness?
 11. We are holding hands?
 12. When I am not able to reach you?
 13. You look at other men (women) with obvious interest?
 14. I reach out to touch you?[8]

If you have a hard time expressing your feelings, writing on one topic for ten minutes might be easier. Then spend ten minutes sharing and dialoguing on what you and your husband have written.[9]

The Emotional Male

There are many important elements required for a strong marriage besides good dialogue. One of them is that your husband should also feel fabulous—about himself, you, and your marriage. Many women have a tendency to forget that men are human beings too and have needs just like their own.

Simply because your husband has male organs and yours are female, don't make the mistake of thinking he has a different set of emotions as well. He's been taught not to show them— that's the only difference.

Little boys are taught early by their mothers (and fathers) not to cry when they hurt. "Big boys don't cry—you don't want to act like a little baby, do you?" And with that admonishment, the male child builds a concrete wall so that he does not show, and oftentimes does not consciously feel, his emotions. As he grows older, his mind turns to the larger details of life: "How am I going to earn a living?" How he feels is pushed into the background because there are too many other things to think about.

But underneath it all, he's sensitive. He hurts. He feels. He needs love and acceptance. He needs to be made love to. He needs to feel special—he needs to cry, to laugh, to play, to be in your thoughts, and to be surprised occasionally.

He's also vulnerable, but in a different area than you are, reveals Cecil Osborne in *The Art of Understanding Your Mate.* "He is vulnerable in such areas as his capacity to earn a living, (hold a job, win success), in the area of sexual performance, and in any area which challenges his male image. Because he is so vulnerable, a wife can emasculate a man by holding him up to ridicule or berating, criticizing, or challenging him. He can be provoked into a towering rage or caused to retreat into the silence of his own loneliness by a remark which he perceives as an attack or a challenge."[10]

As an example, one of my friends related how angry and defensive her husband became over what she thought was a casual remark. My friend suggested that her husband allow his secretary to carry more of his responsibilities at his office. Instead of perceiving the comment as a concern for his welfare and health, her husband translated it as criticism and rejection; he then acted in a defensive manner.

Of course, none of us enjoy the feeling of rejection. Conscious awareness of your mate's needs and sensitivities can eliminate some of the rough spots. It's tough to feel fabulous if you know your husband is feeling less than that.

Right now, go over the following list and check off those areas in which you feel your husband is sensitive:

1. Capacity to earn a living
   a. Degree of success in his profession or occupation
   b. Amount of money he earns
      (1) Ability to keep up with determined standards
2. Sexual performance
   a. Quality
   b. Quantity
3. Being ridiculed or criticized
4. Being challenged or attacked

Unless your husband is a most unusual man, you have probably checked off every one of the items. Now make every effort to avoid those areas in conversation, unless you can talk about them in a sincere, positive way. Always remember, your husband needs his ego built up by you, as much as yours needs to be elevated by him.

Overlook His Faults

If you want to elevate your mate's ego, you'll heed this excellent advice that came from Thomas Fuller, when he said: *Keep thy eyes wide open before marriage; and half shut afterwards.*

Keeping your eyes half shut means you've become mature enough to overlook the unimportant. It also means you have the wisdom to know when and how to handle the important issues.

Do learn to overlook unimportant trifles, though, such as what day Aunt Martha came to visit. He says: "It's the fifth of March." You say: "It was the fifteenth!" Does it really matter who is right? Of course not—because it doesn't affect your life or your marriage in any way. Don't argue over those unimportant issues.

Do learn what is important. When you've had your feelings hurt—that's important. And it must be dealt with. For example, if I'm hurt over a sharp response from Tom, and I get angry inside, instead of snapping back as I would have in my first marriage, I wait. I talk to Tom about it later, when I'm less emotional. Then I tell him I was hurt and why. Notice: I tell him *I* feel rejected or whatever *I* feel. I don't say, "You made me feel . . . ." When I accuse him and make him responsible for my feelings, he is cornered, and there is excellent ammunition for an explosive argument. You can see that it accomplishes nothing constructive.

Feelings are extremely important to talk about. Many people aren't aware of their feelings and need help to identify them. Don't confuse *how you think* with *how you feel*—that spells t-r-o-u-b-l-e when you're trying to communicate.

Before you blurt out anything, love must always be your first consideration. Honesty, though important, must always be used with discretion, for honesty cannot erase the hurt you may cause your husband. As you can see, wisdom and maturity are vital ingredients for a successful, joy-filled marriage. And even though we may not feel wise, I have found that if I ask for it, ". . . God gives wisdom and knowledge and joy. . . ."[11]

So, with your eyes half shut, at forty-plus, one way to feel fabulous is to make the most of those precious years ahead by overlooking your husband's faults and concentrating on the good things about him. As a rule, your husband's faults will be far outweighed by his good qualities. That's where you'll want your focus.

Learning to focus on understanding your mate can be made easier by following the ten commandments for wives that Cecil Osborne outlined in his book *The Art of Understanding Your Mate.* They are:

1. Learn the *real* meaning of love.
2. Give up your dream of a "perfect marriage" and work toward a "good marriage."
3. Discover your husband's personal, unique needs and try to meet them.
4. Abandon all dependency upon *your* parents and all criticism of *his* relatives.
5. Give praise and appreciation instead of seeking it.
6. Surrender possessiveness and jealousy.
7. Greet your husband with affection instead of complaints or demands.
8. Abandon all hope of changing your husband through criticism or attack.
9. Outgrow the princess syndrome.
10. Pray for patience.[12]

(Ten commandments for husbands are also listed in Dr. Osborne's book.)

Now read over the ten commandments again. Make a large red check mark by the ones you feel will benefit your marriage. Diligently and consciously work to make those part of your daily living patterns.

As you have seen, a good, solid marriage that will withstand the storms of time, kids, finances, emotions, and other unexpected interruptions revolves around not taking each other for granted in any way.

Probably the first question to pop into your mind is, "Is it realistic to think that I can love my spouse for better or for worse, yet not take him for granted?"

Yes you can! But it involves *awareness, commitment, communication, good leadership, and overlooking each other's faults—* all smothered in an abundance of top-quality love. The next chapter will show you how to apply these principles. But for now, in order to help you develop a more fabulous marriage at forty-plus, complete the following assignment:

Assignment: **Achieving a Fabulous Marriage**

1. Renew your commitment to your marriage. Really think through what your marriage means to you. Discuss this with your husband.
2. Discuss with your husband his leadership role as God intended it. Is he comfortable with it? Are you?
3. Develop communication skills. Read: *Communication, Key to Your Marriage,* by H. Norman Wright; *The Secret of Staying in Love* and *Why Am I Afraid to Tell You Who I Am?* by John Powell.
4. Become aware of your husband's emotional needs.
5. Make a conscious effort to overlook your husband's faults. Think before you speak!
6. Become aware of the ways you take your husband for granted.

What's so remarkable about love at first sight? It's when people have been looking at each other for years that it becomes remarkable.

11

How to Be a Fabulous Wife (and not Take Your Husband for Granted)

A good wife ... is far more precious than jewels.[1]

In chapter ten we set up some basic principles that can keep a marriage fabulous at forty-plus or any age. Now we are going to see how to put these necessary elements into practice.

You may be thinking that all of this seems pretty one-sided—that the responsibility for perfecting your marriage is falling squarely on your shoulders. I hope that it won't be a one-sided affair—most husbands are open to a better marriage but are hesitant to initiate the change. He'll be more receptive, however, if you take a diplomatic approach, than if you attempt to shove a whole new plan for change at him. Do be gentle and remember two things: Most people do not like change, and *you can change no one except yourself.*

Do remember—if your mate isn't receptive, start making changes in your own life and this may bring changes in your mate. Initiate your own changes with sincerity and love, and you'll be pleasantly surprised at the results.

The Risk of Communication

"Listen to all the conversations of our world, between nations as well as those between couples. They are for the most part, dialogues of the deaf."

I repeated Dr. Tournier's quote because I want you to really think about the tragedy at which it points. Every human, man or woman, has a deep desire to be heard and understood. But communication is not a cut-and-dried subject whereby I can give you Step One, Step Two, and Step Three and whammo, you have instant dialogue.

Our ability to communicate involves the depths of our being. As you grow and remove the destructive emotions we talked about in the first part of this book, your ability to communicate on a deeper level will grow. As I mentioned, you must love yourself enough to be willing to let people see you as you really are.

The unfortunate thing is that the inability to communicate freely brings loneliness, and loneliness increases our inability to communicate. You must consciously step out of that destructive circle and take action. Right now, I'll help you to understand the five basic steps to communication that John Powell has explained fully in his book *Why Am I Afraid to Tell You Who I Am?* which I encourage you to read in its entirety.

Gut-level Communication

1. *Gut-level communication (emotional openness and honesty)* must never imply a judgment of the other. If I judge you, I have only revealed my own immaturity and ineptness at

friendship. But I can say, "I am ill at ease with you," for that tells you *my feelings;* that is emotional honesty. I also have not implied that it is your fault. I take full responsibility for my feelings. It is simply a report of how *I feel.*

2. *Emotions are not moral (good or bad).* Experts in psychosomatic medicine say that the most common cause of fatigue and actual sickness is the repression, or denial, of emotions. We must rid ourselves of the notion that certain emotions are "bad." They are factual; the feelings of jealousy, anger, sexual desires, fears, and so forth, do not make me a bad person. *What I do with them* is the important factor.

3. *Feelings (emotions) must be integrated with the intellect and will. We must experience, recognize, and accept our emotions fully. It does not imply in any way that we will always* act on those emotions, for that shows immaturity. It is one thing to feel and admit to myself and to others that I am afraid, but it is another thing to allow this fear to overwhelm me.

4. *Emotions must be reported.* If I am to tell you who I really am, I must tell you about my feelings—whether I will act upon them or not. If I am to open myself up to you, I must allow you to experience, or encounter, my person and tell you about my anger and my fear or whatever. Too often we fear that others might not think well of us if we tell them how we feel. However, we fool no one, for those feelings generally are transmitted on an unconscious level, and our friend "feels" what we fear to say.

5. Most of the time, *emotions must be reported at the time they are being experienced.*[2]

In a nutshell, dare to express your feelings to the person with whom you are involved. The rules apply to anyone, but specifically, we are talking about a husband-wife relationship, where feelings are continuously generated. A marriage relationship cannot be a close, personal one without an interaction of feelings being communicated.

That doesn't mean you'll only be talking about your feelings, but it does mean you will *include* talking about your feelings, rather than avoiding them.

Right now, make the attempt to learn the difference between expressing opinions and feelings. I'd like you to do a little role playing with yourself. Role playing is acting out a specific situation, such as this one that I'll give you. This is your role: Your husband has just insulted the fabulous omelet you have cooked for him, and you feel hurt. What will you tell him?

1. I'll let it pass as though it didn't happen.
2. I'll get angry and tell him to go to Jim's Diner for his next breakfast.
3. I'll insult him back with a belittling remark.
4. I'll say: "I really feel hurt because you didn't like the omelet. Makes me feel rejected and like I don't want to fix you another one."

Score yourself 100 points if you picked number four. Number one builds resentments inside of you that will pop out sooner or later. Numbers two and three are both explosive and can start an argument. Number four deals with the problem squarely—gets it over with and out of the way. Your husband knows he hurt your feelings. You didn't accuse him of anything. The air is cleared.

Don't Let Marriage Become a Habit

Balzac said: "Marriage must conquer the monster that devours it—its name is habit."

Yes, there are some habits that must be formed, and some that must be broken—and eliminated. If only we could devour the habit of taking each other for granted!

Too soon after the wedding bells ring, marriage falls into a monochromatic routine. Patterns are formed that only awareness can break. One pattern that develops in almost every marriage is expecting our mate to do the simple, everyday things that make us comfortable. And more often than not, we forget to acknowledge when he has done them for us, and taking our mate for granted becomes routine.

The mountain of habit builds according to the number of things we take for granted: the weekly paycheck from the man who goes to work when he'd rather be out fishing; the trip to the store to pick up milk or a loaf of bread during rush hour; mowing the lawn instead of enjoying a game of golf; a washer repaired when he's so tired he's ready to drop; your car taken in for repair or thoughtfully filled with gas; a helping hand while making the bed; dinner preparation made easier because he chopped the onions and stirred the sauce; the table cleared off.

On and on the list goes. There are a hundred and one things a couple must do to function as a team—and a hundred and one ways to take each other for granted.

Instead of taking for granted all those things your husband does for you, develop the habit of acknowledging and thanking him. That includes lovemaking. It also includes the smallest incidental things, such as handing you a glass, or the toothpaste. Learn not to take him or anything he does for granted.

The woman with an ageless attitude is acutely aware it's the little things in life that count. Those are things that make life worth living. And there's a reward. A husband adores doing things for the wife who appreciates him and tells him so often.

Right now, take the time to reflect. How many everyday things do you take for granted? List them:

List at least ten things you'll want to thank your husband for:

1.   9.
2.   10.
3.   11.
4.   12.
5.   13.
6.   14.
7.   15.
8.

List one thing you'll want to thank your husband for *today:*

Make Him Feel Special

I once read and have always remembered that the cry of every man's soul is for admiration.

Showing the man we love the admiration he craves and deserves is a simple action—but one we fail at most often. Marriage is the place where most of our needs should be filled. When those needs are met, there's a willingness from both partners to generate good feelings in each other.

Making your husband feel he's important is not only done with words, but by your attitude and actions. To bring freshness and love to your marriage, try snuggling up on the sofa with that man of yours. Add a little background music and soft lights—a good setting for genuine communication (not conversation). It is a time to share your disappointments, dreams, and goals. And maybe iron out some problems while you're both relaxed and receptive.

Or have a simple candlelight dinner for two at home, with a fire crackling in the fireplace. Even a Sunday afternoon picnic can be fun with a loaf of bread, some cheese, and your favorite beverage. All you'll need is a babbling brook.

If you're innovative, you might come up with a plan similar to Karen's. She arranged to kidnap her husband from his office on a Thursday afternoon. After tipping off the office staff to her plan, Karen blindfolded her husband, led him out to the car, and drove him to the airport. There, she handed him two tickets (saved for, for months out of the grocery money) to Phoenix for a long weekend of golf, swimming, relaxing in the sun, delicious food, and lovemaking.

Karen's husband adored the surprise and the special attention. "I felt like king for a day. We've recaptured the closeness that was fading. It was great to be alone with Karen—away from the kids and all those pressures on weekends."

Any weekend away can be meaningful. It doesn't have to be elaborate or expensive. A camping trip with sleeping bags, if you both enjoy camping, can be a precious time. And it doesn't have to be a whole weekend. An evening alone can be special. The important part is that you schedule your lives so that the two of you can be alone—to share your love. *Make it a point to take time to be together!*

Oftentimes, Tom and I will drive over to the marina to spend a quiet evening together on our boat, *The Challenger*. Our dinners there may simply be hot dogs and potato salad. The food isn't as important as having our time together, with no phones, doorbells, or kids interrupting. We can talk or just relax—it's our time.

Sometimes *I* suggest going to the boat; other times Tom does. Being together is what it's all about. Many women are not used to being the assertive one when it comes to arranging activities. I know many wives who sit back and pout because their husbands seldom think of things to do.

But the woman who is Forty-Plus and Feeling Fabulous about herself and her husband doesn't wait for him to take the action. She arranges for picnics, walks, a game of tennis, theater tickets, dinner reservations, or calls her husband for a luncheon date occasionally.

I realize there's a danger in this, and you might be thinking,

"Yeah, but I get tired of planning everything all the time!"

What does it matter who plans as long as you're doing things together and he's agreeable? He has enough on his mind, coping with his occupational frustrations while earning a living. *The important thing is to be together.* Again, it's a positive attitude that makes the difference.

You can't always be together, of course, but there are little things you can do to let your husband know how important he is to you. I like to keep my marriage fabulous by sending special greeting cards to my husband at his office. No special occasion—just to let him know he's on my mind and that I love him. I also send him red carnations on our anniversary: one flower for every year we've been married.

Sending flowers is just one way to fill your husband's need for admiration. One wife I know (not yet forty-plus) stays sensitive to her husband's needs by having a standby sitter. After a particularly rough day at work, Jim called home about 4:00 P.M. He just couldn't face the kids, the noise, and confusion. "Jill, see if you can get a sitter and meet me at The Madison at 5:30, okay?"

If Jill had shrugged and said, "Oh, gosh, Jim, I'm too tired. Why don't you just come home?" Jim's reaction next time might be: "Well, Jill's not interested. I'll stop and have a couple of beers with the guys."

Being available isn't the only way to show love. Pride in your husband is a priceless attitude. Look for ways to sincerely praise him—privately and in front of family and friends. You'll make him feel ten-feet high when you say things like: "Did you notice the nice job Tom did on the lawn today? It sure looks great!"

If your compliments are sincere and natural, your friends will love hearing you extol each other. No one likes being around the couple who put each other down.

And it's no joke when a husband is laughed at or ridiculed for sharing a farfetched dream. Many a husband would like his wife to be his best friend, lover, and companion. The way to become that special person is by developing the ability to listen, to encourage, and appreciate. Remember: *Friends never give unasked-for advice or criticism!*

You can still be a friend even though you have been married to the same man for twenty years or more. You've probably settled in with the same sense of comfort as wearing those scuffed old slippers, and the habits have almost become engraved in stone. But it's not too late, nor is it too early, to change. Right now, take the time to make the following evaluation:

1. When was the last time you and your mate did something for fun together?
2. What kind of things do you plan to make your husband feel special?
3. How do you show your husband love?
4. How do you make your husband feel appreciated?
5. When did you last admire your husband?
6. When did you last compliment your husband?
7. Go back over questions one to six and jot down a positive action you will take this coming week in each area.
8. Plan a surprise for your husband this week.
9. List other areas you want to improve upon.

What If My Marriage Is Worn Out?

At forty-plus, many women are thinking they would like to get out of their marriages. If this is where you are, I'd like you to turn that attitude into a challenge to create a better marriage, instead of leaving your marriage behind. There are many marriages God did not create in heaven. But most of them are worth salvaging. Divorce is a painful experience, as you will see in chapter thirteen. Those of you who have not been through one have no doubt been close to a friend or relative who has. You've seen the emotional turmoil that is caused by breaking apart two people who have been together in one body called marriage.

Marriage is a vital part of life. But marriage must be managed. Taking the relationship for granted, instead of building, building, building, is what causes marital rot.

I wish marriage-management courses were mandatory in our schools, or at least before couples are issued a marriage certificate. If we had a clear realistic picture of a marriage relationship in the early years, perhaps the divorce rate would be far less today.

We all know the divorce rate is staggering. And it doesn't matter whether a divorce occurs in the early or later years—it causes great pain for the children. You may think that a divorce at forty-plus will not affect your adult children. Wrong! I remember how devastated my twenty-eight-year-old friend became when her parents' thirty-year marriage ended abruptly. I don't know when I've seen anyone more emotionally rocked than she as she watched her parents pull apart.

There is no time when divorce does not take an emotional toll. I don't know how bad your situation is (I hope it's very good, but I know many are not). I do know there is help available.

To give you hope, I want to share a real love story about my sister, Judy. Tom and I hadn't even unpacked our bags from a ski trip to Europe when a frantic phone call came from Judy, asking if she could come to visit for a month. My heart sank as I learned of the tragedy stirring in her marriage of fifteen years. There was divorce and more heartache than words on paper can aptly describe. Little Jamie was eight; Joey, ten. Joey moved in with his father; Jamie stayed with Judy.

Knowing she'd have to become a part-time mother, Judy applied for a job and was hired on her first interview. That was the beginning of a new life. She had no way of knowing that the real-estate firm that hired her was owned and managed by a devoutly Christian man who held prayer meetings every morning. (If you remember, our religious upbringing was almost lukewarm.)

Her employer not only held prayer meetings, he held a deep

concern for the struggles within each person in that office and practiced the kind of Christian love that helped each one to grow.

This isn't the story of an overnight healing of a marriage. It was a slow, painful, sorting-out and growing process for both Judy and her former husband that took three years. During that time Judy grew from an insecure, dependent girl into a strong, loving, giving woman.

With a group of other women, her last act of singleness was a six-week trip to Europe and the Holy Land. When Judy returned, her former husband was waiting to reunite in marriage.

Judy, her husband, and two children have been a family for over a year now and are working as a team. Even though I personally had seen no hope for that remarriage to become a reality, God had. But both Judy and her husband were willing to make the changes required to accomplish that.

There are many ways to make the changes that create a strong marriage—before it crumbles. I hear glowing reports from couples who have returned from a marriage-encounter weekend. Information about these marriage-enriching sessions can be obtained through most any church, Catholic or Protestant. Couples are taught during the forty-four hours away from home how to dialogue about the things that generally are carefully sidestepped in everyday living. After the initial forty-four hours, couples attend monthly meetings in their own area.

These weekends are not just for marriages needing rejuvenation, but for those who want to keep their marriages fresh and exciting. One young couple in our church, married only a short time and still beaming, returned even more in love after a marriage-encounter weekend.

Yokefellow groups meeting weekly are another way to develop awareness and make changes. As I mentioned in the introduction, these groups usually have about ten people who meet for no less than thirteen weeks—generally much longer, because the small group is such a healing, loving experience.

Your own city or town will have other marriage counselors; many churches also offer help.

There are precautions to take if you choose counseling at random from the phone directory or other sources. I urge you to find out ahead of time who the leader or counselor is and what his philosophies are. Unskilled or self-centered counselors can cause more havoc in your life than you already have. Before you attend, ask questions and evaluate responses from those people you talk with.

When I need help, I feel it's important to find Christ-centered leadership or counselors because it's important to me that our focus come from the same source. For example, if I'm trying desperately to keep my marriage together, but the counselor leans more toward divorce than marriage saving, our focus is different.

In addition, there are "me"-centered counselors and philosophies that can also distort your values. That is why I feel caution must be taken.

Another reason why I prefer Christ-centered counselors is that they know God is the Great Healer and through praying and changing, healing will come.

However, even though you believe in God's healing powers, you cannot passively sit around and wait for God to make the changes in your marriage. You must initiate and carry out the action. Then the healing of your marriage can take place. Prayer gives you the strength to go forward.

I believe that healing can come in just about any situation. I like to remember what God told Moses in those early days on the mountain: "... the place where you are standing is holy ground."[3] Too many of us are like cows in a pasture—we think the grass is greener on the other side of the fence. But God said that *where we are standing is the holy ground.* It's not in another marriage.

I hope you cherish your marriage as I do mine. But, if it's less than fabulous, do invest the energy to turn your marriage into the kind of relationship that is vital. Always remember that your attitude plays a crucial part in how you see your marriage.

Assignment: **How to Be a Fabulous Wife**

1. Learn and practice the five rules for gut-level communication.
2. Practice ways to break old marriage patterns that indicate you've taken your mate for granted.
3. Learn and practice ways to make your mate feel admired. Concentrate on one special way this week.
4. Evaluate your marriage. Dare to discuss the evaluation with your husband. If your marriage is in trouble, seek competent help immediately. The shame comes in not asking for help, not in needing it.

A woman must be a genius to create a good husband.

BALZAC

12

Developing Fabulous Sex

I am my beloved's, and his desire is for me. Come, my beloved. . . . I will give you my love.[1]

The last two chapters have been devoted to creating a fabulous marriage now that you're forty-plus. In this chapter we're going to discuss a very important part of marriage: sexual intercourse. All of the attitudes we have discussed up to now are basic to developing fabulous sex.

Sex does not begin and end in bed. Sex begins with your a-t-t-i-t-u-d-e toward your husband while you're lying together in the morning and your thoughts of him during the day, when you happily look forward to being together again.

One very important attitude you must be sure to communicate to your mate is this: *Your husband wants to know you need and desire him as much as he does you.* There's nothing more exasperating to a man than a passive sex partner. As one man said: "A passive wife is as exciting as making love to a log."

Meanwhile, greeting your husband as he comes through the front door after a hard day's work is one of the most important nonpassive acts of the day. But many women don't realize the importance of this gesture. This simple act is not only significant, it's symbolic.

168

Many European mothers train their children to run to cheerfully greet their fathers at the door when they return from work. These wise mothers know the importance of making their husbands feel needed and important the moment they enter the house after a hard day's work.

Many men feel neglected when their greeting consists of only a casual, "Hi," as though they had been gone only a moment. All too often this passive attitude is carried into the bedroom, where the same lack of intensity is applied to sexual attitudes.

Every man looks for a visible sign of welcome and being loved as he walks through the front door. He needs to know he is an important part of his wife's life.

"But how can I express this to my husband if I haven't been used to doing it?" you may be asking. You will need to make a conscious effort to change your actions and attitudes.

Attitudes

Do attitudes really affect my sex life? Yes!!! Yes!!! Yes!!! An ageless attitude at forty-plus is as important in your bedroom as it is in any other room of the house. We've been talking about attitudes all through this book, and now we've invited your attitude into the most intimate place of your life—your marriage bed.

I know about wrong sexual attitudes, because I was raised with them. Many of us who are forty-plus were taught by mothers who had puritanical attitudes toward sex. Those attitudes may have been passed on to you verbally or in an unspoken way.

Unless you've made a conscious effort to become aware of those damaging attitudes, they could be invading your marriage bed. And really, there's no room (even in a king-size bed) for Mom and Grandmom's outdated, useless sex attitudes.

But I didn't know that when I was first married at the tender age of twenty. After a strict upbringing, the signing of a marriage certificate failed to automatically license me to enjoy a sexual relationship with my husband. I thought of sex as dirty and a bother. Those attitudes were harmful to both my eager, young husband and not-so-eager me.

To a husband, negative sex attitudes translate as r-e-j-e-c-t-i-o-n. I might add, that happens at forty-plus as well as in the early years.

I once read that it takes about ten years to erase those Victorian attitudes—so if a wife is twenty when she marries, she might be thirty before she begins to enjoy sex. From that point on, her husband better be prepared to keep up with her.

I found that to be true in my own life. But before I reached that stage, I had Christian counseling and worked very diligently to change my attitudes through prayer and constant attitude awareness.

Right now would be a good time to take inventory of any secondhand puritanical attitudes. Check off the ones that apply to you:

Sex is dirty.

Only men enjoy sex.

Women aren't supposed to enjoy sex.

Nice women don't enjoy sex.

Sex is for man's pleasure only.

Sex is for reproduction only.

Women never actively desire sex.

Only men should initiate sex.

Only men reach orgasm.

A man's penis is dirty.

Physical Problems

Let's deal with the problems that are of a medical nature before we discuss orgasm. At forty-plus, during and after menopause, you may experience a dryness in the vaginal tissues that comes from the decline in estrogen. Because this condition can make sexual intercourse very painful, you'll want to keep a lubricant, such as a petroleum jelly, by your bedside. There's almost nothing more distracting than trying to make love in an atmosphere of painful friction.

This is a serious problem and should be brought to your doctor's attention. Dr. Sheldon Spielman (who addressed the problem of osteoporosis in chapter five) often prescribes estrogen cream for his menopausal and postmenopausal patients who are *not* on estrogen therapy.

A small amount of estrogen cream inserted into the vagina once or twice a month usually takes care of the problem. Dr. Spielman feels that even a woman who cannot take estrogen because of the cancer danger to breast and uterus, can use a small amount of estrogen cream, even though it is absorbed systemically. One application of cream is equivalent to about one estrogen tablet.

Vaginal dryness is a common problem during the forty-plus years, and you won't feel fabulous as long as the problem persists. Don't be ashamed to admit you have it—your doctor will be sympathetic.

During these years you may have the tendency to shove sex aside. Don't! Sex must be practiced and perfected if it is to be enjoyed, like any other fine art.

Tom and I have discovered that during the infrequent times our sex life does slack off for one reason or another, it takes more frequency and practice to get back in the swing of things again so that we both enjoy it to the fullest.

Being forty-plus is a good excuse to feel fabulous. But it is not a good excuse to ban sexual activity or fulfillment with your mate. In the excellent, informative *The Menopause Book,* we read: "It is clear that during and after menopause, an interesting sexual change often occurs: women become more erotic. Some older women have more sexual fantasies, masturbate more frequently, and want sex more than when they were young. Rather than fading away with the decline of estrogen, their sexual desire increases."[2]

Could it be that it has something to do with the empty nest? Does life become more conducive to romance because there is more privacy and freedom? It *is* nice not to worry about kids knocking on your door at the crucial moment. With the children gone, your husband can again begin to see you as his lover, rather than the mother of his kids.

And speaking of kids, we can score one more for menopause and being forty-plus—because this is the time of life when you no longer have to worry about unwanted pregnancies. But menopause can be a tricky time, and there are a few mid-life babies to prove it. Be sure your fertility has turned to sterility before you discard birth control. That judgment is best made with your own doctor. Then relax and enjoy your fabulous sex life.

This is a good time to take inventory of any physical problems that may be keeping you from enjoying sexual intimacy with your husband.

1. Dryness
2. Pain (describe)
3. Other

Orgasm

Once the physical problems are out of the way, our thoughts can turn to another annoying problem. This one is especially frustrating to many women and their husbands. I'm talking about the inability to achieve orgasm. Like menopause, it's a subject many would rather sweep under the rug than admit they have.

But you can't sweep it under the rug and expect to experience the ultimate in pleasure with your husband. Many women have never experienced orgasm but are ashamed to talk about it.

Many experts feel the problem is a psychological, not a physical, one. According to Dr. Ed Wheat, in the informative book *Intended for Pleasure,* "The problem may be rooted in the past, even before marriage, but psychological causes can seldom be exactly pinpointed, and the only purpose served by seeking something in your past is to find someone or something on which to place the blame."[3]

Once you realize that your nonorgasmic state is only temporary, even at forty-plus, you are free to begin your attitude change.

Attitudes do play a large part in sex, as in other areas of your life. In one of my Yokefellow groups a forty-plus woman admitted to the group that she had never experienced orgasm during her twenty-year marriage. After some attitude changes toward herself and her husband and a releasing of her puritanical views of sex, she began to experience the long-awaited, magical orgasm. Her courage to share with the group gave other nonorgasmic women hope for themselves. It's never too late to achieve a climax. Unless you give up!

Dr. Wheat and his wife, Gaye, speak to the problem and give specific instructions for overcoming nonorgasm in their book *Intended for Pleasure*. They remind women that one of the first steps in obtaining orgasm is desire. "If you desire to have an orgasm because you know it is your right, your provision from God, and because you want to keenly enjoy the most intimate times with your husband, then there is no reason why you cannot experience an orgasm. It will come."[4]

One of the ways that is extremely helpful in achieving orgasm is through the use of your mind. In Dr. David Reuben's book *Everything You Always Wanted to Know About Sex but Were Afraid to Ask,* he says, "The only thing that stands between any woman and an unlimited number of orgasmic experiences is about two pounds of tissue—the brain. The decision to have a sexual climax is not made in the vagina—it occurs at the other end of the body."[5]

Even though it occurs in the mind, simply telling yourself you want to have an orgasm while you're making love is not the right mind-set—not then. You can benefit by learning to fantasize while making love, not worrying about having an orgasm.

Perhaps we should stop to define *fantasy* to avoid confusion and get rid of any negative, preconceived ideas. Webster says fantasy is: "the free play of imagination . . . a fantastic notion . . . the power, process or result of creating mental images modified by need, wish, or desire . . . to portray in the mind . . . daydreams."[6]

But why would I be telling you to daydream while you're making love? Because your thoughts intensify all the feelings that send messages to your brain.

And the free play of imagination? Just what does that mean? It means that to achieve or intensify orgasm, your mind must be as active as your body, or more so. You must think about what is going on—the pleasures you are receiving and ones you are giving. Concentrate on every touch and anticipate each move, both yours and his. Think of new ways to bring your husband pleasure and to intensify his orgasm.

Think, too, about how much your husband wants, desires, and craves your body. And you should have the same yearning for his body. Right then, you are his entire world and he should be your entire world. Wonderful things are happening—you are sharing in the best you each have to give; you are communicating with your entire body, mind, and soul.

Lack of orgasm can be a failure of total communication. If you're thinking about tomorrow night's dinner party at Jane's and what you're going to wear, your focus is wrong and you'll likely be minus an orgasm. An orgasm requires the full attention of your mind, body, and soul.

You may think that fantasies only belong in kinky relationships. The word itself raises all kinds of fantasies in your mind. There's nothing kinky about telling each other of your desires for each other, or how good you make each other feel, or describing those feelings during sex.

Fantasies come in all qualities. They can be gentle, clean, and pleasing. They can be as pure as Snow White and as sparkly as Tinkerbelle. They're yours—you are the creator.

Of course, it's extremely important to work with your husband to develop a better sex life. Chances are, if you've been nonorgasmic, your husband feels guilty and inadequate and assumes some of the responsibility. You'll want to relieve him of that guilt as quickly as you can.

Not reaching orgasm is only one problem connected with an unsatisfactory sex life. Another common problem is ignorance of your own body as well as that of your husband's. Do you know the names and functions of your own female organs? Do you know the names and functions of your husband's male organs? Do you know the mechanics of an orgasm?

This isn't a sex manual, so I urge you to run, not walk, to your nearest library or perhaps your own bookshelves and find the best book you can that will explain all the things you don't know but need to. Sex is no different from anything else in which you want to become proficient. First, you must learn all you can about it.

Right now, answer the following questions. Include your husband in the discussion and have a handy reference book to help answer your questions.

1. What is an orgasm?
2. How does it come about?
3. Ask your husband how you can make his orgasm feel more fantastic.
4. What don't you understand about your husband's body?
5. What don't you understand about your own sexual body?
6. Have an honest talk with your husband about sexual fantasies. How does he feel about them? How did you react to the section on fantasies?

Give Your Husband Pleasure

You've no doubt heard it said many times that happiness in itself cannot be found; it is a byproduct of giving of yourself. Sex is no different.

Sex becomes good for me when my husband is sexually satisfied in every way—when I can make him feel as though he has given me the ultimate in what he has to give.

Or in the words of Gaye Wheat, "It begins with the attitude of thinking about him instead of being preoccupied with myself. It includes looking for ways, all the time, to help him and please him."[7]

When you concern yourself with your husband's pleasures, you'll be in close tune with his feelings and realize that you, at forty-plus, have no monopoly on change. Your husband, too, is forty-plus and going through changes. You should be aware that sexual changes are occurring, although there is not necessarily a decline in sexual activity or desire.

According to several medical reports, by the age of fifty, a man has a slower sexual response. He no longer has instant erections, and it takes him longer to have an orgasm.

If you're an observant and sensitive wife, you can help your husband adjust to this change by understanding his fears and being helpful and patient. It's an excellent opportunity for you to take a more active sex role, if you've been used to being a passive wife.

In the opening of this chapter, I mentioned that making love to a passive woman is as much fun as making love to a log. Many men feel this. Why do women allow themselves to become logs? Puritanical attitudes have pushed many a woman into a sexual-martyr role. That is, a woman knows it's her duty to give herself to her husband. However, she is not actually giving herself. She is giving only one small part of her body. When a wife inactively lies there, it makes a man feel as though he has used her. He not only feels guilty, but resentful.

There are some wives who *do* understand how their husbands feel. The little story I'm about to tell is rewarding for most men because they would like more aggressive wives "bedside," at least part of the time.

Frieda and Walter are a forty-plus couple who have a fabulous sex life. If you ask Walter what makes it so special, he'll light up and say: "It's because of Frieda. I can hardly wait to get home from work in the evening to see what Frieda has thought up. I'm really a lucky guy: first, because Frieda enjoys our sex life; and second, because it seems as if every day, she spends a little time thinking up fresh, exciting ways to be intimate with me. Our sex life never gets stale—she's a very creative woman."

Creative sex! That's what Frieda has developed in her marriage and that's what every guy wants—a wife who enjoys him and sex enough to look forward to it, to plan it, and to take the initiative frequently.

You, too, can make your sex life adventurous. There are more sex manuals available than I could possibly list. Many of them give illustrations that leave nothing to your imagination, such as the bestseller *The Joy of Sex* by Alex Comfort. Only the application is left up to you. Don't hesitate to study and use these manuals with your husband. Besides being useful guides, the manuals can be quite stimulating to look at. Planning your sex life together is one more way to add some concrete to your foundation, as we discussed in the marriage chapters.

But marriages are not all romance as we well know, and sometimes it's too easy to fall exhausted into bed at night, especially if your jobs cause a lot of tension. That is often the case with Tom and me. But one of the things that Tom enjoys is when I gently arouse him after he's been asleep. Then we make love—and fall asleep again.

Perhaps your husband won't always respond in the middle of the night; he may be too tired or sleepy and say so. That's the time your ageless attitude and self-love must be strong enough to not register his refusal as rejection. Understand it for what it actually is—fatigue and the need for sleep. He still loves you!

And lovemaking doesn't always have to be in bed at night. One of the mistakes too many forty-plus couples make is falling into a deadly routine—same place, same time, same position, same bed.

Instead, use your imagination and pretend you're his mistress. Greet him in a lovely, sheer negligee when you know you are going to be alone. Or meet at a motel in another town. Plan a weekend away and make love as though it were the last time.

I love what Jason Towner said in his book *Jason Loves Jane* (*But They Got a Divorce*), because it has tremendous depth and reflects how we take each other for granted, even in lovemaking. These are words I hope I never forget:

> Our kisses were too short because we thought we had forever.[8]

How many times do we make love as though we'll be making love again tomorrow? All too often, most of us would have to confess. So we just don't put everything into it today! This is another faulty attitude—one that blocks sexual fulfillment.

The rest is up to you. In chapters one through three you learned about several tools with which to remove destructive attitudes and replace them with positive ones. If you are hung up on some puritanical sex attitudes that are blocking your love life with your husband, remember that God saw everything that he made and behold, it was very good.[9]

I'll close this chapter with a quote by Charles R. Swindoll, from his excellent book *Strike the Original Match,* in which he further reinforces that "God personally and caringly created the human body, so that it might be stimulated, aroused and able to enjoy to the fullest, in marriage, the complete expression of sexual delight."[10]

Assignment: **Developing Fabulous Sex**

1. Concentrate on finding any destructive sex attitudes and replacing them with positive, pleasure-giving attitudes. Use the same flush method and other techniques for change given in the first three chapters.
2. Become aware of any physical problems that are bringing pain to sexual intercourse and seek medical care this week.
3. If you are nonorgasmic, read chapter seven in *Intended for Pleasure* by Ed and Gaye Wheat. Work on overcoming the problem. Seek professional help if necessary.

4. Use your imagination and creativity during lovemaking. Be persistent and determined about achieving orgasm.

5. Find ways to give your husband sexual pleasure. This week, plan one special time for lovemaking and tell him about it ahead of time so he can be thinking about it all day, as you will. Then plan the setting, what you will wear, how you will look, and most important, how you will give your husband exceptional pleasure. Use illustrated sex manuals if you can't think of new techniques yourself. During the day, build up the same kind of enthusiasm and excitement that you did when you were dating and you looked forward to seeing your lover. Show him you are genuinely happy to see him; be demonstrative when he arrives home. If this all seems phony, playact it until it becomes a natural part of you.

Part V
Surviving a Divorce

13

Do You Really Grow Through Divorce?

*For if you forgive men their trespasses, your
heavenly Father also will forgive you.*[1]

We've talked about building a fabulous marriage, but I realize all marriages are not salvageable and some have already dissolved. One of the enemies of the woman who is forty-plus and trying to develop an ageless attitude is, ironically, divorce.

In chapter five, we talked about menopause and now I want to introduce you to a subject that is relatively new, at least in public attention getting. The male menopause, often referred to as the male climacteric, is not experienced in the sense that women experience menopause.

Paula Weideger, in her informative book *Menstruation and Menopause,* describes the *climacteric* as "the transition made during a period of fifteen to twenty years between the biological state of middle age and that of older age (roughly spanning the period between one's mid-forties and mid-sixties). Climacteric changes, therefore, may be observed in all body tissue and body systems in members of both sexes. Within the context of the climacteric, menopause is only one event taking place in the female body."[2]

Weideger explains that "there is no clear-cut period during which the male sex hormones drop in production and realign at a new, lower level. There are, therefore, no male symptoms which are by-products of profound hormonal readjustment. (Men, of course, retain fertility throughout their lives.) Males do not experience a biological event that symbolizes the arrival of age, but they do most certainly experience climacteric changes, among which is the decrease of potency, along with the aging process of tissues and bodily systems that affects every part of the body."[3]

Then just what are the signs of the male mid-life change? There are many. According to *The Menopause Book,* the physical symptoms are: "irritability, fatigue, restlessness, anorexia, insomnia, often indecisiveness. Depression may be perceived as hopelessness, sadness, or pessimism, or may be expressed in physical symptoms."[4]

As I mentioned before, sexual problems are common at mid-life. Career changes and change of life-style may also be symptomatic. But divorces, extramarital affairs, sexual problems and depression are the leading problems according to Dr. Barrie Anderson.[5]

Because the male mid-life change has been ignored by medical science until recently, many men bump into mid-age completely unprepared for the thud.

And considering that the "male menopause" and yours may be happening simultaneously, it's no wonder that so many divorces occur during the mid-years. This time is even more complex than adolescence, with hormonal changes and personality changes taking place in you and your husband. Sometimes the immediate solution to these perplexing problems seems to be divorce.

Is Divorce an Acceptable Solution?

If divorce is a solution to one problem, it may well be the cause of several others. The Bible, church, and society all make authoritative judgments, and what they say may influence the way we handle a divorce. Let's take them one at a time.

The Bible leaves no doubt in our minds where God stands on divorce. Jesus said, ". . . What therefore God has joined together, let not man put asunder."[6] Because of that and other biblical teachings, it has been easier to live unhappily (also a sin) than to cope with guilt brought about by divorce.

Next is the church. Many churches would rather not acknowledge that today divorce has become a reality and divorced people need to be ministered to. They become judgmental, rather than extend a much-needed hand in the healing powers of Christian love and companionship.

Jim Smoke, leader of divorce seminars nationwide and author of a book I highly recommend, *Growing Through Divorce,* says that in his personal counseling, many have told him their divorce has caused them to reexamine their relationship to God. They want to be closer to the church and make a commitment to God, but the church does not always make it easy for the divorced person to feel comfortable, or to experience forgiveness.[7]

> Many people who experience divorce while involved in church and religious life are asked to move their membership and families elsewhere. Others are removed from future leadership roles in the life of the church and are imprisoned in the pews as a permanent penance for their misdeeds.
>
> We don't have to tell them (the divorced) it's wrong. They're already suffering tremendous guilt because they know it is. What we need to say is, "How can we the congregation help you?"[8]

To further draw attention to the problem, *Moody Monthly,* a Christian family magazine, recently captured the reader's eye with the provocative title, "Does Your Church Treat Divorced People Like Criminals?"

That title immediately tells us that the unacceptance of divorce in many churches is not past tense but an ongoing struggle. Cynthia Scott, writer of that dynamic article, challenges the churches to stand by their members who are confronted with "financial changes, emotional grief, altered social relationships, loneliness, sometimes unwanted independence, and the prospect of raising children as a single parent."[9]

The church is changing its attitudes slowly, and if you talk with other "singles-again," you'll be able to find a church that does welcome you with open arms. My own church, Columbia Presbyterian, in Vancouver, Washington, is one of those. I realize you can't all attend a church near Portland, Oregon, but do look in your own area for such a welcoming church.

Even though the church is slow to change, much of secular society has come to view divorce as an acceptable means of handling a deteriorating marriage.

Still, "one-time marrieds," have a tendency to be somewhat judgmental of divorce—and if not of divorce itself, the woman who has been divorced. Terms such as gay divorcee, the merry widow, and swinging single are used by people who have never experienced divorce and know not the deep pain of separating from someone who has grown to be part of you.

In spite of all the judgmental attitudes that are present in our society, the fact remains that last year an estimated 1,182,000 marriages in this country ended in divorce. Double that number and you have 2,364,000 hurting, lonely women and men.[10]

It is these hurts that we will be concerning ourselves with on the next several pages. Healing can be a long or short process after a divorce, *depending on your attitude and determination to proceed with your life.*

One of the first attitudes you must concern yourself with is your feeling about divorce. Believing that a divorce is necessary does not always erase the feeling of guilt for dissolving a marriage.

As Christians, we know that God forgives divorce, although He does not recommend it. However, most of us still feel guilty because we've broken one of God's laws. Let's balance the scales right now. Even though you are divorced, you don't have to feel guilty the rest of your life. Jesus went about forgiving the sins of several women in Bible times. One was the woman of Samaria who had had five husbands and was living with a man to whom she was not married.[11]

If you are divorced or are in the process of divorce do not burden yourself with unnecessary guilt. Your life is complicated enough without that added burden. If God is quick to forgive us, surely we can be gracious enough to accept His forgiveness and go on with our lives.

Let me be quick to add—if you should try to justify all your wrongs on that premise, you'll break yourself. You can't repeatedly break God's laws without paying the consequences in some way.

The ability to forgive yourself is one of the attitudes that will keep you from dwelling on past failures that prolong misery. Use your failures to learn from—never as a hitching post. You can be sure your wounds won't heal until you've removed the thorn of guilt.

Once you've forgiven yourself, don't think of your divorce as a failure, but rather as a successful decision. And more important, don't think of yourself as a failure. This time can be the threshold of a successful new life.

Shortly after my divorce, while I was still carrying the thorn of self-pity, my teenage son Tim had to remind me that all was not lost. With his arm tightly around my shoulder, he tried to cheer me with: "Remember, Mom, this is the first day of the rest of your life."

But when the wounds are deep and painful, it's difficult to think that the days are going to be better. However, life does bring healing, slowly, day by day, inch by inch. In my life, God did keep His promise when He said, "I will restore health to you, and your wounds I will heal. . . ."[12]

So Your Prince Charming Turned Into a Frog?

It's not easy to look at yourself and see a success when the world has shattered at your feet. I was barely forty-plus when THE SEPARATION came. Fortunately, I had gone back to work a couple of years before. My job as secretary to the public relations manager in a large corporation offered me some financial security and some self-identity—and I was thankful for it. But my emotional-security problem was more complex than that.

Like many women in my age group, my identity revolved around being Mrs. Somebody's Wife—in my case, the wife of a banker, a very prestigious position in any community.

But my identity was suddenly yanked away by the loss of a husband who no longer wanted to be married. It was a frightening realization to face my life as a single person. I'd have been a total wipeout if my long involvement in Yokefellows hadn't emphasized having Christ as the center of my life and, the use of positive attitudes.

Now, six years later and happily married again, as I sit here on our boat, moored on the Columbia River, with snow-covered Mount Hood towering to the east, and the lush green hills of Portland to the south, it's difficult to realize I was that weak, frightened person. I was almost demolished by the breakup of a marriage to a man I no longer loved and with whom I had so little in common. Yet—that was me. And it happens to many women who are forty-plus and not expecting it.

After I quit feeling sorry for myself and stopped wallowing in self-pity, the extreme pain gave me the determination to become a whole person again, and not to rely on being Mrs. Somebody's Wife.

It didn't take me long to figure out that with my shattered self-image, I didn't have a lot to offer the kind of man I'd require as a husband. I knew I'd have to be as mature and together as he was, or I'd be searching for a long time. I also knew I wanted to be married again—someday.

After the buckets of tears ceased to flow, it was time to pull my act together and get on with living.

Being addicted to the list method of problem solving, I set about to evaluate myself to see where I was, emotionally and physically. There were emotions to reverse, my health to rebuild, and my future to plan.

I began the list. I was scared. Scared of what?—of being on my own for the first time in my life. (If I'd been age conscious, I'd have been real, real scared.) I'd always lived with another adult. Worse yet, I had to take full responsibility for every decision I'd make.

Loneliness was my constant companion. My mother had died of cancer a few months before. I hadn't fully recovered from that loss, which was the first close death in our family. My father and sisters were 1,200 miles away. Married friends tend to disappear when a divorce occurs, leaving you feeling even more isolated and scared.

I turned to my church for help, but the minister was having personal problems of his own. I tried another minister, who helplessly tried to soothe my wounds with, "Remember, God loves you." I didn't feel loved. I felt alone and lost.

That was when my prayers pleaded for healing of my entire body, mind, and very tired soul. I read every positive, soul-building book I could find. I saturated my mind constantly with positive thoughts about myself and life. In addition to the Bible, James Allen's *As a Man Thinketh* became a great source of strength.[13]

Next on my list of mental things to fix up was financial security. I'd grown up during the Depression and my parents' concern about lack of security rubbed off on me. Even though I'd been promoted to a top-paying position as an administrative assistant in a larger department, had a couple dollars in the bank, and was able to continue living in our warm, comfortable home with Tim and Tobi, I worried. I had everything in the world going for me; yet I lacked faith.

As if being scared and worried weren't enough, my first winter alone was the "pits." If God's intent was to make me strong, He did it in every way possible! Winter was the worst I'd ever experienced. Of course, having grown up in southern California, a heavy thirty-degree frost was a bad winter!

For example, driving on ice became a real challenge. My country home was at least two steep, winding miles from the paved highway. Part of it was gravel, with a sharp incline that was impassable in bad weather without a four-wheel drive, which I didn't have.

For almost three months, intermittent snow and ice covered our hill. After work, I'd stop in town at the last service station to have chains put on my tires so I could drive home.

In the morning, I'd stop at the same station to have the chains removed so I could drive the snow-plowed highway the eleven miles to work. Once the chains punctured my tire. Another time, the battery was dead in the morning. I went back to bed and cried myself to sleep. Thank God for a sympathetic boss with unending patience!

If it's possible to feel helpless and lost—but determined—I did!

Deliberately, I worked on each item on my list—again— taking the top-priority one and channeling all my efforts into accomplishing it. It took weeks, sometimes months. But I was persistent and successful. I prayed and prayed and prayed. I was determined to rebuild a self-image that would take me through snow, ice, flat tires, and dead batteries.

I was able to weather the divorce more easily because of three people: Louise, a faithful friend who was also in the throes of divorce; Emily, a happily married co-worker who added stability to my life; and Alma, a devout Christian woman whom I shall always love and appreciate.

Alma had been my son Tim's teacher. During that time her husband died and we drew closer. God became our common denominator. Alma became my close friend, counselor, and private pastor during those long months of struggle during the divorce. She was always there when I needed her.

Many hot tears flowed as we prayed together, bound in love by God's Spirit. She'd gently remind me of the biblical message: "For the husband is the head of the wife . . . ."[14] If this divorce was his decision, I'd have to accept it.

It was through Alma that Louise and I learned about Saint

Luke's Episcopal Church near Seattle. There, the Spirit penetrated, soothed, and healed our exhausted souls.

As I grew stronger in my faith, I grew stronger in myself. Accepting my new life was only one of the many things I continued to work on as my list of growth-to-be-accomplished grew shorter.

Growth can come in unexpected ways. One of the most memorable experiences I'll always cherish is the Mother's Day my daughter, Tobi, invited me to go hiking with her. An avid hiker and mountain climber (unlike her mother), she promised it would be an easy two-mile hike to the lake nestling securely in the mountains. Against her advice, I wore tennis shoes and carried my heavy purse. Tobi carried the food and water.

It was beautiful and serene in the Cascades, with the ferns fresh and green from the rains and the fragile trillium in bloom. But the rocks penetrated my thin soles; my purse felt like a trunk. I tired easily but Tobi gently pushed and I went on, a bit at a time. I was on the verge of anger—I didn't like to push myself. But Tobi knew I could make it and didn't give up. We trudged on.

Near the final bend, I was determined to turn back! Tobi assured me the worst was behind us; the path would be level and easy around the bend. Around the bend the path *was* level; the worst *was* behind me; and the clear, blue lake, breathless and majestic as she promised.

If I had turned back, I would never have known the worst was behind me; the effort would have been wasted. That was a lesson I'll never forget. That experience came during the most painful struggle of divorce. It gave me a promise that life would be sweeter tomorrow. "... Weeping may tarry for the night, but joy comes with the morning."[15]

Friends like Louise, Emily, and Alma and even the understanding of my loving children helped me through the dark times. I believe that those three women were a key to my recovery and regaining of self-esteem.

If you are in the throes of divorce or the doldrums that follow a divorce, if it's at all possible, find a close woman friend who is also single. You can be a precious comfort to each other during this time of readjustment and feeling alone, rejected, and confused. You need someone you can trust, share, cry, plan, and grow with—someone who has the same moral standards you do—someone you can pray with.

Before we go on to the next chapter, I'd like those of you experiencing divorce to take the time to evaluate where you are. As you do this, remember that it's your *attitude* toward a given situation that is harmful. As soon as you can reverse that attitude, you will have won another battle.

Assignment: **Do You Really Grow Through Divorce?**

1. The following is a list of emotions with which most newly divorced women grapple. Read them over, then check those that apply to you. Be aware that each involves attitude:

   Financial insecurity
   Shattering of a self-image that was based on your husband or husband's position
   Depression
   Fear of living alone
   I-can't attitudes
   Feeling sorry for yourself
   Inability to earn a living
   Feeling too old to remarry
   Feeling like a reject
   Feeling like a failure
   Scared of the dating game
   Worried about your social life
   Worried about your sexual needs

Once you have gathered your attitudes together, you'll be able to sort them out and handle them constructively. The next two chapters will walk you through the stages of divorce and show you how to grow instead of grope.

Each stage has its own meaning—life is a step-by-step process. Each step has its meaning.

PAUL TOURNIER

14

The Challenging Stages of Divorce

If you do not forgive men their trespasses, neither will your Father forgive your trespasses.[1]

There are no stages of divorce that are pleasant and fun, but each stage must be dealt with if you are to get back to the place where you like being forty-plus and feel fabulous about yourself and your life. And it *is* possible; I can vouch for that. Again, your attitude and determination play the major role in how your life is going to turn out.

I remember one divorced young woman who had a tremendously poor self-image and negative attitude about life. When Tom and I were to be married, she was excited and happy for me. But her comment was "Well, you must have 'something' to find a man like Tom." The "something" she referred to was my tiny bank account and country home. I tried to explain to her that having material things had nothing to do with it. It's a positive attitude that attracts a man with a successful, positive life. Negatives attract negatives. Positives attract positives.

Because of that simple law of nature, you'll want to release all attitudes that attract negatives and apply the principles of positive thinking that you have learned throughout this book.

We'll take the stages of divorce as I experienced them and work them through so that you'll come out with positive attitudes. You will actually *grow through your divorce, not just go through divorce.*

Before we begin, let me urge you to seek out other divorced Christian people who meet weekly to work out their problems and uphold each other emotionally. Louise and I floundered through mostly on our own and learned about these support groups after we'd worked through the problems. We would have given anything to have known of their existence during our struggles.

Mourning

You don't have to dress in black for a year, but mourning is a necessary stage of divorce. Writing in his helpful book *Creative Divorce,* Mel Krantzler says:

> Next to the death of a loved one, most of us find divorce to be the most traumatic experience in our lives. When we consider that we refer to our mates as "my life," "my right hand," or "my better half," we should not be surprised that separation from that mate produces reactions in many ways identical to those which an actual death can set in motion. Divorce is indeed a death—a death of a relationship; and just as the death of someone close to us brings on a period of mourning during which we come to terms with our loss, so too a marital breakup is followed by a similar period of mourning.[2]

Mel Krantzler, author also of *Creative Marriage* and *Learning to Live Again,* goes on to say that such denial is dangerous. The mourning must take place whether or not you deny or suppress those feelings. But its healing powers will not be effectively utilized unless you do allow them to surface. All the feelings of that loss must be accepted. The mourning process is important because it provides a way for you to ventilate all your conflicting feelings, which will eventually lead to your growth as an independent person.[3]

In my own case I remember clearly, speaking of my former husband in the past tense, as though he had actually died. I was surprised to find myself referring to him that way, not knowing then that the mourning process was essential. It was after that psychological "burial" of my marriage that my life did take on new direction.

Another reason for the burial is this very important one. If you plan to marry again, the old marriage must truly be buried. I have seen second marriages where the former spouse is brought into the conversation far too often to indicate a proper burial has ever taken place.

Throughout this book we've talked of removing the old before the new can take hold in our lives. It is to be accomplished by the use of the flush method and by substituting positive attitudes. In a divorce it is also important to flush away the old before something new and wonderful can be born. If you are having trouble releasing your former spouse and marriage, use the familiar flush method, described in chapter two.

Now use this checklist to see if you've experienced the mourning period.

1. Resentment and bitterness toward your former mate have turned from twenty-four-hour obsessions to occasional spurts of anger.
2. Less time is spent complaining—more time is spent on problem solving.
3. You see old friends again.
4. You are making new friends.
5. You begin making decisions based on your own interests and pleasures, not your former spouse's.
6. You don't lump all men into one category.
7. You realize you aren't the only divorced person.
8. You accept your divorce as a solution, not a failure.[4]

Build a New Self-Image

Besides becoming aware that you must have a mourning stage, you'll want to beware of those first feelings of rejection that register: "No man could possibly want *me!*" They are extremely dangerous and must be recognized immediately. When you feel like that (and most women do), you're liable to grab the first male who comes along.

The first male relationship to come along in my life was a disaster, but I could see only through fog-coated glasses at first. He was a handsome airline pilot who was charming, divorced, with no children. His wife had divorced him many years earlier when she learned of his unfaithfulness. He had become an alcoholic. (I learned all this later.)

Fortunately for me, he seldom kept his word, and I became disgruntled with the relationship. I was lucky. Some women are not. Building a positive self-image is probably one of the surest ways to help guard against falling for the first man who asks you to dinner. Low self-esteem can be hazardous to your health, even though the federal government hasn't declared it so. You'll be jumping off the barbeque grill right into the hot coals if you don't recognize those defeating attitudes right off.

It's important to become aware of your own feelings and the needs those feelings arouse. Remember back in chapter one, when we discussed personality as *parent, child,* and *adult?* Never is a woman's *child* more vulnerable than after a divorce. The *little girl* in her needs love desperately—so desperately, that a woman will often be blind to the male con artist who has charm she can't resist. But in reality, he is interested in money. Many women have been left heartbroken and minus large amounts of money by the pro who preys on their vulnerability. These gigolo types understand the psychology of women only too well.

According to one woman who was a victim even after discovering her scheming lover was married, her addiction to him was too strong for her to pull away. She continued to lavish her money on him, knowing in her mind she was in the hands of a professional con artist. But the emotional needs of the *little girl* surpassed all logic.

These men have a magnetic, satanic charm that is difficult to resist. (Some women have even been known to give up their children for them.) The con artist is an unscrupulous vulture who knows the widow or newly divorced woman is easy, unsuspecting prey for him and his voracious hunger for money.

Of course, the majority of men are not con artists, but you'll still want to examine your relationships closely. Remember, too, that men who are newly divorced suffer the same feelings of rejection as you and may want to rush into a premature marriage. For those of us who are forty-plus and have been married more than half that time, marriage has created a protective cocoon, and the world can be a cruel place as you enter it as a single-again.

Right now, sit quietly and contemplate where you are emotionally. Check those items that best describe you.

1. I feel unattractive.
2. I'd feel lucky to go out with any kind of man.
3. I don't have anything to offer a man.
4. I can't compete with all the pretty young girls.
5. I'm too scared to think about men at all.
6. I hate men.

Sexuality

Emerging from that marital cocoon and being naive about the single life can bring many laughs. The divorced woman must be aware of the current social trends. There is an acceptance of sex for the single-again. That doesn't mean you have to participate, however. The choice must be made by you.

One of the funniest experiences a group of recently single-again women and I had came at the first singles-club potluck dinner dance we attended. It had taken us days and days of accumulated courage to make the decision to go. The event was sponsored by a large church in Seattle, and we thought it might have some credibility. After all, it was a church!

Wrong! The room was packed with men and women of all ages. There was no lack of dancing partners. Around eleven, the hall began to empty as couples disappeared. My friends and I looked at each other and wondered about the mass exodus. We soon realized what was happening. Couples were pairing off for the night, or perhaps the weekend. The dance was simply a "meat market"—a term that also shocked us. That was a rude awakening—one of many.

After that, we made a pact: If we went someplace together, we'd return together.

Divorce will present you with a true test of your moral values. Do you say yes or do you say no? The Bible clearly states that sex out of marriage is forbidden. Yet, I heard a minister-counselor say that sex out of marriage is okay if no one gets hurt by the relationship: that is, if both people understand what that relationship means, and one doesn't think it means love, while the other uses it for sexual gratification.

But that's not what the Bible teaches. Religious and parental teachings create great conflicts within the divorced woman who continues to have the same sex drives she had in her marriage. Although sex for the single woman has become the accepted, rather than the exception today, the Christian woman must consider this: When she breaks God's laws, she breaks herself as well, in some way.

Sex outside of marriage is a topic many Christian writers would rather not tackle. But Harold Ivan Smith has done an excellent job of setting out the problems of sex for the single-again in his book *A Part of Me Is Missing.*

Sexuality is a very controversial subject within the church— well, actually it's not even controversial—it's mostly ignored! But anyone living in the real world knows that it is a crucial concern and issue.

To ignore the needs of the single-again when you are married is easy. But when you are suddenly thrust into the situation yourself, you become acutely aware of the sexual conflicts and problems divorce brings.

One of the ways to deal with the problem is to examine your reasons for needing sex. Harold Ivan Smith says that "sexual relations are a deliberate stroking of the ego as well as physiological response . . . . The need in single-agains for intercourse often is more emotionally motivated than physiological. The warmth of cuddling, hugging and being held makes sex sensational and affirming. And God designed it that way."[5]

However, warns Smith, "the single-again can easily become overly dependent upon sex. Emphasis is placed on sexual *relations* rather than sexual *relationships.*"[6]

> Sex becomes either a pain-killer that gives temporary relief from a sense of failure or personal undesirability, or a mood-elevator that counteracts chronically low self-esteem . . . they get no lasting satisfaction after all; they feel good about themselves, reassured for a short time after each "fix" but within a day or two, or even within hours, the bouyant mood dissipates and anxiety, despair and self-contempt creep back in.[7]

Temporary sexual gratification can come from casual sex, but when the pleasure fades, you again have to look in the mirror and face your values. So whether your needs are simply to be held close, or your sexual desires run high, your values will have to be determined before you find yourself in a horizontal position. When your blood runs hot and your brain has turned to putty, all your biblical and moral convictions will be forgotten until after the moment of ecstasy.

Ideally, the growing Christian woman will strive to turn over her sex drives to God and pray that He channel those sexual cravings toward greater control and maturity.

I read someplace that cold showers still work, but I hate cold water!

I don't see anything wrong with talking about these very real problems with the man you date. If you tell him ahead of time what you will or will not do, the cards are on the table. He may be as relieved as you to know he doesn't have to play sexual games.

However, some men are quick to make it clear that they expect sexual intimacy as part of the dating game. It was those demands that caused one woman to duck out on the problem altogether. Even though she yearned to be held, cuddled, and more, she could not yield to the need. Rather than have her strict moral standards frustrate her, she dealt with her sexual desires by not dating at all. She threw herself totally into a new career and allowed her bitterness toward men to grow. The problem is, you can't run away from your own sexuality and be happy. It must be dealt with, not shut out.

As a contrast, another single-again accepted a kindly gentleman's invitation to visit his apartment one night. Lisa's need for sexual intimacy ran high and she found herself in a bed she hadn't consciously planned to inhabit. The next morning Lisa's sexual needs seemed trivial compared to the guilt that consumed her. She felt cheap, dirty, and used. With all the other complexities of divorce, Lisa didn't need multiple infractions too. After her painful recovery from an acute loss of morality, Lisa quickly put her priorities in order.

Both women found there is no quick, make-a-list method to solve this important need in their lives. What I've implied—celibacy—does not sound realistic to me or to you. But the Bible is definite. Can the Bible be bent to meet the social mores of our times? I wish I had an answer for you; I don't. But I would have felt guilty to bypass this important sexual problem in this book, because I know how real it is.

And so do many of your ministers; they can offer counsel. Jim Smoke, author of *Growing Through Divorce,* offers seminars and workshops across America. Perhaps at your request, your church could arrange to have a workshop for singles. And be sure an article goes into your local newspaper inviting *all* singles to attend.*

Examine yourself now. Honesty is very important. Unless you deal squarely with your sexual needs, you'll not make the decisions yourself—you'll be forced into them. It's not possible to feel fabulous at forty-plus if you're being forced into sexual roles that you'd rather not play. Answer the following questions and then decide how you will handle your sexual needs.

1. Do you believe sex outside of marriage is wrong?
2. What does having sexual relations mean to you?
3. Do you believe in sex without love?
4. Do you (or would you) engage in sex because of social pressures?
5. Do you believe intimacy is wrong if two people love each other?
6. If you are dating, are you peaceful about the way you are handling your sex life?

Resentments and Forgiveness

Handling your sexual urges is only one of many adjustments you'll be required to make as a single-again. Forgiving your former husband rates high on the list of "musts."

"But the rotten bum left me and took off with his pretty, young secretary! I'll never forgive him. I hope he . . ."

You might be justified in feeling that way, but the woman who is forty-plus and again wants to feel fabulous, will not accomplish her goal by holding on to negative attitudes of bitterness and resentment. They will harm her. It's wasted energy. Those attitudes are not going to change anything, and they certainly won't erase the hurt. You must forgive him.

"Why do I have to forgive him when it feels so good to hate and say awful things about him?"

---

* For information about Divorce Recovery Seminars, write to Jim Smoke, 395 Loretta Drive, Orange, California 92669 or phone 714-633-7320.

Because what goes into your mind and body must come out—in some way. If a destructive thought (hate, bitterness, resentments, unwillingness to forgive) goes into your mind, becomes an emotion, and is kept, it will fester, and you'll have your own Mount St. Helen's volcanic eruption.

It's no accidental choice of words when people say things like, "I can't stomach that man," then bend over with ulcerating pain. Or, they may say, "That's really eating away at me," as they gulp down the Maalox. And oftentimes, it is doing just that—eating away their insides with unhealthy acids their stress is causing. Many times your own vocabulary can give you a clue as to what is happening inside your body.

Another good reason for giving up bitterness and resentment is your need for estrogen during menopause and after. When your body is tense and under stress, the adrenal glands turn off the estrogen and concentrate instead on fighting off tension. Then you have double trouble, as we discussed in the menopause chapters.

At best, hate, resentments, and bitterness will sap your energy. And right now, you need all your energy to develop those positive attitudes that will make you feel fabulous again.

Don't let the bitterness from a divorce cause you to take two steps backward now. Don't allow the root of bitterness to grow within you. It will spread and blot out your gentle, feminine spirit.

Perhaps every spouse is bitter after a divorce. I was, for a while. As soon as I saw the direction I wanted my life to take, my feelings changed. I hoped that my former husband would find a good life and marry someone who could make him happy. I felt sorry I had unintentionally let him down in many ways through my immaturity. Today, I still want the best for him.

Unfortunately, it takes some women several years to completely release their former spouse. Some never make it. Bitterness and resentment make it extremely difficult when children are involved, even when they are adult children. It's painful enough for your children to see the two people they love most, divorce—and even worse for them to have to see you inflict lingering pain on each other.

The whole idea of divorce is to end the relationship—cut the ties—let go of each other—*in every way!*

If you consider that bitterness and resentment form one emotional tie that still binds you together, you may be more willing to release those negative emotions and forgive him. When I recognize something like that, I get so mad at myself for letting a negative emotion control me, it gives me the determination to make a change right there and then.

Another way to make that change is through prayer. When I resist a change that needs to be made, I pray that God will give me the willingness to make that change.

Not only in divorce, but in every area, forgiveness is part of a healthy woman's life. Not only is it commanded by God, it is required by our body, mind, and soul, if we are to be healthy and vital. Daily, we need to forgive and be forgiven.

No matter what your destructive attitudes are, they certainly are not worth carrying any longer. That's why the Bible has so many graphic teachings on forgiveness. Here are a few:

> . . . whatever you bind on earth shall be bound in heaven, and whatever you loose on earth shall be loosed in heaven (Matthew 18:18 RSV).

> For if you forgive men their trespasses, your heavenly Father also will forgive you; but if you do not forgive men their trespasses, neither will your Father forgive your trespasses (Matthew 6:14,15 RSV).

> . . . "Lord, how often shall my brother sin against me, and I forgive him? As many as seven times?" Jesus said to him, "I do not say to you seven times, but seventy times seven" (Matthew 18:21,22 RSV).

> . . . forgive your brother from your heart (Matthew 18:35 RSV).

Right now is a good time to empty those troublesome emotions down the drain. Just flush them away and feel the burden

204 SURVIVING A DIVORCE

being lifted from your heart. Substitute the kind of brotherly love that Jesus commands us to have for our neighbor.

1. Bring into awareness the emotions of bitterness and resentment. Write those here:

2. If you have not dealt with these emotions, you might want to write a long letter to the man you have divorced. Tell him all your hurts and how much you hate and resent him. Write everything you feel. Get it all out. As soon as your letter is complete, tear it into a hundred pieces and burn it. Release the emotions at the same time. Then fill the void with positive attitudes.
3. Practice the art of forgiveness. If the old thoughts come back, keep emptying them until they no longer return. Be sure to replace them with loving thoughts.
4. If it seems natural and comfortable, tell your former husband (in person, by phone, or by letter) that you are sorry if you have hurt him in any way. Then wish him a happy life.

As you can see, it is necessary to face and deal squarely with each stage of divorce as you come to it. None can be bypassed if you are to grow through your divorce into a woman who feels fabulous about life. There are still some important stages of divorce that we will look at in the next chapter, but for now, we'll stop for the assignment that will help you accomplish an ageless attitude.

Assignment: **The Stages of Divorce**

1. If you haven't mourned the death of your divorce, go back and sort it all out and bury the marriage. Do not sweep it under the rug. Handle all the emotions one by one, using the flush method, and replace them with positive attitudes. Read *Creative Divorce* by Mel Krantzler and *Growing Through Divorce* by Jim Smoke.
2. Work on building a new self-image. Find the emotions that scare you. Work on them one at a time until you feel positive about yourself.
3. Make a decision on how you will handle your sexual needs. If you need direction, seek professional help.
4. Concentrate on ridding yourself of all bitterness and resentments. Forgive yourself and your former spouse. Use the flush method and replace all negative emotions with positive ones.

15

Is There Life After Divorce?

*. . . goodness and mercy shall follow me all
the days of my life. . . .*[1]

While you're working to eliminate the immediate problems that have been brought on by divorce, you'll also have to think about your future. Career plans must be made. Even though you may not need to work for financial reasons, it's still crucial to set some goals and go after them.

Keep in mind that at forty-plus you still have lots of years ahead in which to develop a career. And being divorced should give you the incentive to put some enthusiasm and thought behind it.

But many women do not have enthusiasm and zest for living at forty-plus. They appear to have burned out. We all know women who have been divorced from wealthy businessmen. Preoccupation with the job market is not their prime concern. They live in beautiful homes, travel extensively, and dress with elegance as they compete with other fashion-conscious jet-setters.

Many times, however, these jet-setters are withering away as the loneliness becomes unbearable. When depression becomes a companion, they hide out at home, refusing to answer the phone or to socialize. Sometimes excessive liquor blots out the elegant poise and grace they have carefully developed.

Why? What's missing from these lives that appear to have it all? A life direction.

Perhaps you find yourself in the same boat as these women. I don't mean an excess of money—I do mean, with no goals for your life. As you work your way through the maze of obstacles caused by your divorce, look for creative ways to spend your time. The sooner you can take your mind off yourself, the faster you'll resume living a normal life.

As I said before, when my divorce came, I was fortunate to be working for a large corporation. It was a company that offered many opportunities for advancement. I took advantage of all the relevant programs offered. I also took college courses at night to advance my skills, or develop new ones. I approached my job as a career—as though I would be working for the rest of my life. In the six years I worked for that company, I learned a variety of skills and felt confident I could qualify for many good-paying and worthwhile positions.

If you aren't working, one of the things you'll want to consider is going to college to learn a new skill, or sharpen up on old ones, or just for the sake of learning.

Or, you might consider volunteering your time. Many schools have programs through which you can help teach children who require special attention. Also, the many refugees who have recently come to this country need help learning to speak English and adjusting to American life. You can help them while you help yourself.

Right now, check off the items that apply to you:

1. I need to find a job now.
2. I must learn new skills in order to earn a living.

3. If already working, I will learn more skills so I can progress in my job.
4. I want to go to college and learn a new skill before going to work.
5. I do not have to work. I will consider volunteer service.

Evaluate the One You Let Go

When you've been recently divorced, the emotional incompatibilities present in your former marriage are still fresh in your mind. It's extremely important not to forget what they are, so I'll be asking you to write them down a bit later. Time has a way of erasing the unpleasantness of a former marriage.

The *only* reason you'll want to make a note of the conflict areas is so that you will not repeat the same mistakes again. One of the requirements of an ageless attitude is that you learn from your mistakes, remember? I'll be telling you that many times, because it's extremely important.

Too many women remarry and haven't the slightest idea why their first marriages crumbled. Oh, sure, they can see the symptoms because they are usually obvious. But treating the symptoms is a poor cure—you have to get down to the heart of the matter. And that's what you'll be doing when you honestly evaluate where the emotional hang-ups were.

You'll need to realize that, usually, you are 50 percent of the reason your marriage shattered. Once you've taken that responsibility, don't waste time brooding about it. Use the information to grow.

You'll find many of the reasons are going to be unfulfilled emotional needs. When your emotional needs are not being met, there is big trouble. While you're evaluating how your former mate didn't meet your needs, think about the other side of the coin, because if your emotional needs weren't being met, you can be sure his needs were not being met either.

That's why it's so important to pick a mate with whom you

are compatible. Someone once said that a man takes longer to choose a suit of clothes than he does to take a wife. Too many times, picking a mate is based on the wrong reasons.

I was determined I'd pick a mate for the right reasons the second time, and by the time I met Tom, there wasn't a doubt in my mind about the kind of man I wanted to marry. I'd had my list made out for about three years. I knew the qualities I wanted and needed and the kind of man whose needs I could meet.

Your list of emotional needs will not only help you understand why your marriage ended, it will prepare you for a successful future. When you are dating someone you see as a potential mate, evaluate your personalities so you will know if they mesh—or thrash—before your relationship becomes too emotionally involved.

Right now, go over the following checklist. Read it through carefully. Then go back over it and check off those areas that apply to you. Add to the list. Use it as a guide to evaluate your needs and the needs of your former mate.

1. He is the silent, inward type, and you need someone who can communicate freely. He may be the serious type, and you need humor, gaiety, and fun.
2. You love to dance; he didn't even try to learn.
3. You are adventurous in foods; he'll eat meat and potatoes, cooked one way.
4. You like to talk and leave the lights on while making love, but he likes it dark and quiet.
5. He is negative toward life and people. You are positive and happy and see only the good side. You enjoy being social—having parties and being surrounded by people. He can't relate to people and enjoys solitude.
6. You like to travel. He does too, via TV, in an armchair.
7. You need gifts and flowers to feel loved. He never thinks to send flowers or buy gifts, and you feel neglected.
8. He is a passive fellow—a slow thinker. You are aggres-

sive and quick. When you ask him if he wants a cup of coffee, you want a quick answer—now—not five minutes later.

9. He can't show love and give emotional support when you need it. You need to be touched and held to feel loved.

10. You like togetherness. You'd like him to be your best friend, companion, and lover. He is a loner and scared to respond to those needs. He thinks they are demands.

A Two-Year Investment That Pays Off

A common mistake many women make after their divorce becomes final is to remarry at once. In order to avoid that blunder, let me suggest you do this: Make a promise to a married couple with whom you are close friends that you will not marry again for at least two years—and if, for some reason, you feel you can't keep that promise, you will discuss the matter with them before marrying.

Further, not only will you not marry for two years, you will not allow yourself to become emotionally involved. If you date, it will be casual, for friendship and companionship.

I know you may not like the sound of this, but there are many valid points to back up this advice. First, you are too likely to marry a man with the same emotional makeup as your former mate if you don't give yourself time to grow. I have several friends who say they were too blind and confused after divorcing to see that the second mate had many of the same emotional weaknesses as their first husband. A strong-appearing woman may attract a man who is looking for someone to help carry his emotional load. But the woman may, in reality, be weak and looking for a strong male. But if they rush into a second marriage, they probably will not realize they are headed for the same emotional conflicts they encountered in marriage number one.

Next, it's important that you have a period of time to find

out about yourself. What are your strengths? What are your weaknesses? What do you want to do with your life? Besides a wife and mother, who are you? If you become emotionally involved with another man right away, you won't have the time to stand on your own feet emotionally.

And, you need time to develop into the kind of woman who sees and uses her capabilities to the fullest. Even if your goal is to remarry, it's important to realize that a good marriage partner, ideally, is as emotionally strong as the man she hopes to marry. Once you've been able to overcome your fears, insecurities, resentments, and bitterness, have lived alone for several months, and supported yourself financially, you'll be better able to experience the responsibilities that a husband carries. Wearing his moccasins, as the old Indian saying goes, can make you a more sensitive, supportive wife.

During this two-year period, you'll spend your time rebuilding yourself into the kind of person you never took time to become. You'll consciously work on your lists every day, building those ageless attitudes we've been talking about. You'll develop an attitude of love, trust, compassion, and self-acceptance. You'll concentrate on becoming a strong, self-reliant, independent woman.

It's at this time, if you allow, God will become your unchanging, constant Companion. It may seem morbid to reflect on it here, but nevertheless well to remember: Every human relationship will end. A life built on human relationships only is weak. God gives strength to a life because He is forever.

In time, you will feel capable of living alone, securely, unmarried, financially, as well as emotionally, unsupported. Your relationship with God will grow closer, and you'll discover your strengths come through Him and yourself, rather than through having a husband. Having a husband is a wonderful bonus!

You'll know you are ready for marriage again when you are confident and happy being single. This is the time you'll have something genuine to offer a husband. The diamond in the rough has been cut and polished. Now you can be a strong, supportive marriage partner.

As we conclude this chapter, I hope you feel that there is life after divorce. If you do, these chapters have done their job.

Most women do want to remarry, for life without a husband can be lonely, and ours is a society that believes in marriage. But good marriages don't just happen—and don't let anyone tell you they do. For the Christian woman, prayer for direction and guidance is a must, plus unemotional, objective evaluation.

I want to share a letter that my good friend and former pastor, Vickrey Dougherty, wrote to me before Tom and I were to be married. I had written a glowing report of my new love and anticipated marriage and this was his response:

> The most important thing in any marriage of a Christian is that the mate also be a Christian—not just a nominal one, but deeply committed. Until we give ourselves to Christ so completely that we let Him control our thinking and behavior through His Holy Spirit within us, we are controlled by our own spirits which can be selfish and hostile.
>
> Often, we are unwilling to forgive, accept responsibility, and apologize for hurts we have inflicted on our mate. We too often wait for the other to make the first move. Actually the true Christian will take the first step.
>
> The best guide I can suggest is Ephesians 5:21–33. This is the only workable formula for all truly Christian marriages. Read, pray, and think about it.
>
> It is especially important where the husband is younger than the wife, as in your case. You are to be subject to one another out of reverence for Christ. But it also says that wives should be subject to their husbands. This may seem hard, but it is very necessary in many areas of home life. It should not be too hard for a wife to be subject to a husband who "loves her as Christ loved the Church and gave Himself for it . . . ."
>
> The only husband who can fulfill this instruction is one who is living a life of real fellowship with our Lord, for let's

face it, there are times when a wife is not easy to love, just as there are times when a husband is not easy to love or to be subject to.

In any case, I believe that a home based on the principles given here will be a happy and lasting home.

My friend was right. Even though you may be tempted to shove those words out of sight and claim you'll do it your way, think about them. You may say, "I have the capability of picking the right mate—those words are too restricting." Well, I too once thought that way. But I can testify to their truth and necessity for a happy, loving marriage.

Right now you may not be thinking about a loving marriage because the pains of divorce are too new and deep. Even so, I want so sincerely to tell you and have you believe me when I say that each of you have the capability and potential for the happiness you dream of. I truly want you to feel fabulous about your life right now, about love, and about a future marriage. These things will happen if you take your time to work through all the stages of divorce and not rush into another marriage out of the fears that divorce can produce.

Reread the three chapters on divorce and all the suggested reading. Take the time to complete the following assignment and sincerely make an effort to complete all the other assignments.

Assignment: **Is There Life After Divorce?**

1. Make constructive plans for your life this week. Set goals. They can be changed later, but make some now.
2. Evaluate your emotional needs and those of your former spouse. Make a list and keep it for reference.
3. Make a promise that you will not marry for two years.
4. Make a list of the emotional, physical, and material requirements you'd like in a future husband. (Remember, we usually get only as much as we expect.)

Part VI

Getting the Most Out of This Book

You have done what you could. Some
blunders and some absurdities no doubt
crept in; forget them as soon as you can.
Tomorrow is a new day; begin it well and
serenely with too high a spirit to be
encumbered with your old nonsense.

RALPH WALDO EMERSON

16

Charting Your Course

For I know the plans I have for you, says
the Lord, plans for welfare and not for evil,
to give you a future and a hope.[1]

You may be single, recuperating from a divorce, or happily
married and content. Or you may be preparing for the empty
nest and wondering what to do with your future. Wherever you
are, it's time to make a serious evaluation of your life.

Even though you evaluate your life, it isn't enough. You
must then set new goals and meet them. Some of those goals
may be accomplished with a 21-day plan as we described in
chapter three; others may take 21 years to accomplish. It's not
the length of time that is important—*it is the setting of specific*
goals that gives meaning to your life at forty-plus.

Time Management

We'll be talking about goals a bit later. But first, we need to
discuss t-i-m-e. To get downright philosophical about time,

you'll realize that without it, you cease to be. In addition to eternal life, time is one of the most precious gifts God has given us. Yet, we tend to waste much of it.

A very wise man, Alexander Woollcott, once said, "Many of us spend half our time wishing for things we could have if we didn't spend half our time wishing."

Unfortunately, many people don't even spend their time wishing—they simply spend it in front of the TV set watching soaps and other nondetergents.

In a recent study it was found that the average homemaker watches daytime television an average of three hours daily. That becomes fifteen hours a week, based on a five-day week, or sixty-seven hours a month. On a yearly basis, those figures calculate to about 800 hours—or roughly one whole month, day and night, of solid TV watching.

If that astounds you, you'll be even more astounded to learn that the average family watches television not three hours a day, but six! That makes two solid months out of every year dedicated to watching the tube.

With that enormous chunk of time gone, it's no wonder we hear so many people saying, "I don't have time to . . ."

In order to combat that problem, I'd like you to keep track of how you spend every minute of your time for the next seven days. The object of this exercise is to see where you are wasting valuable time and how you can better use that time to set daily goals, and improve productivity and the quality of your life. This is the chart you will use. Begin filling in the chart now and continue for the rest of the day. Then copy this chart on six pieces of paper and fill in one each day. After seven days, you will see a pattern that will reveal whether or not you are wasting time. If you are, you will want to reschedule your time in a way that allows you to be more productive and also promotes your goal of developing an ageless attitude.

Time	Detailed account of how time is spent
6:00	
6:30	
7:00	
7:30	
8:00	
8:30	
9:00	
9:30	
10:00	
10:30	
11:00	
11:30	
12:00	
12:30	
1:00	
1:30	
2:00	
2:30	
3:00	
3:30	
4:00	
4:30	
5:00	

5:30

6:00

6:30

7:00

7:30

8:00

8:30

9:00

9:30

10:00

10:30

11:00

11:30

12:00*

Here is a sample of how to fill in your time chart:

7:30 up, shower, exercise, makeup, dress
8:00 coffee, read Bible
8:30 breakfast, TV talk show
9:00 TV, phone Leone, coffee & newspaper
9:30 TV, iron, phone Loti, and so forth.

After seven days, make some new charts and record your time schedule as it changes. It will undoubtedly take you a few weeks to develop a more productive schedule, so don't be dis-

---

* This time-management form is used in the Portolese Leadership Institute life-direction class. For more information write: 14915 63rd Avenue West, Edmonds, Washington 98020.

couraged. If the new one doesn't work, change it again. Be open to change. *Having an ageless attitude means being flexible.*

Goal Setting

Finding more time is worthless, however, unless you use it productively. And to do that, you will want to make a practice of setting goals. But first, let's define *goals*—they should not be confused with activities. Busywork is not goal setting. You cannot "do" a goal.[2] Most of our busywork can be classified as *activities*—things we do.

Activities are those things which we do daily. They comprise necessities such as washing the dishes, cooking, running to the market, and so on. We do them easily and regularly.

The difference between activities and daily goals is that the latter achieves something we are not accustomed to doing.

In addition, it is possible to have *daily goals.* For instance, if you have been used to thinking negatively about yourself and your goal is to become aware of and change those attitudes daily, that is a daily goal.

You may also have *short-term goals.* These take longer than a day to accomplish; they may take as long as six months. The daily goals may be the steps by which you accomplish your short-term goals.

For instance, if you decide to change your self-image from that of an impatient, cross woman to that of a gentle, loving spirit who can accept herself, a six-month goal would be appropriate. However, you can clearly see that daily goals are needed to accomplish your short-term goal. You cannot accomplish a goal of any magnitude without working on it daily. For example, to become gentle and loving, your daily goal would include awareness of your negative responses. The second daily goal is to memorize and repeat a Bible verse that emphasizes patience and kindness. Then pray that God will help you be that kind of person.

Short-term goals are a necessary part of a vital life, but you must also have *long-term goals* if you are to feel a sense of accomplishment and satisfaction about your life. Too many people look back with regret and begin numerous sentences with, "If only I'd . . ." or "I wish I had . . ." because they drifted through life without a plan, rather than directing their own life through the setting and attaining of lifetime goals.

Long-term goals are the things you'll look back upon with a sense of accomplishment. These, too, will be specific goals, as are the short-term and daily goals, but obviously will take much longer to accomplish.

As an example, a long-term goal that might be five years away could be a trip to Europe to see where your ancestors were born. Or, you might want a career goal, such as progressing from waitress to restaurant manager or going to college and graduating. Perhaps you didn't graduate from high school and have always wanted your diploma.

While all of these are long-term goals, they are accomplished by setting short-term goals that will facilitate your plan to accomplish the long-range one.

Once you learn to set realistic, attainable goals, your possibilities are limitless. Only your lack of imagination and initiative will hold you back.

The ongoing setting of goals is essential, as is the ongoing development of your ageless attitude. Daily goals and short-term ones designed to establish a pattern of positive thinking will facilitate this long-term goal of feeling fabulous at forty-plus.

Of course, without asking yourself the question, "What is my lifetime goal?"[3] an ageless attitude will be elusive. That is why it is one of the most important questions of your life at forty-plus. You cannot feel fabulous if you don't program yourself for it. *Feeling fabulous is not a free gift.*

Once you learn to understand and set goals, your life will take on the kind of meaning that may have been missing all these years. I recommend that you read Alan Lakein's book *How To Get Control of Your Time and Your Life* for a more thorough understanding of goal setting. This is a vital subject that is well worth the time it will take you to research it.

Right now, take a minute to jot down some tentative goals—ones that are attainable. Remember, goals can always be changed; you aren't tied into them forever. Having a goal is the important part.

Daily goals:

Short-term goals:

Long-term goals:

Organization

Once you capture what was formerly elusive time, and think about goal setting, the next step is organization of your time and household. Without organization, achieving goals can seem like an obstacle course.

An obstacle course is what home was like to two sisters who live here in my own hometown. Pam Young and Peggy Jones are the two self-admitted, desperately disorganized women whose "slovenly lives" suddenly took a slide to fame and fortune.

They tell their tale of trial, torment, and triumph in their earthy, ingenious book, *Sidetracked Home Executives.*

> We were hopelessly disorganized. Our six kids drank out of jelly jars, our husbands had to wear damp socks to work, we were afraid to open the Tupperware in our refrigerators, and we were always locked out, left behind, and overdrawn.
>
> Out of desperation we created a 3 x 5 card filing system for organizing our homes and our lives. In six weeks, we called ourselves "reformed slobs" and decided to share the system with other sidetracked people.[4]

The seminars developed by Pam Young and Peggy Jones are now held nationwide.* I use the 3 x 5 card system for many things in my home and have recommended it to many of my friends. We'll only discuss two uses here, but I suggest you run out and buy *Sidetracked Home Executives* (Warner Books/New York) and use it to organize your home.

These are the supplies you'll need: 3 x 5 recipe box; twenty-five each of white, yellow, blue and pink 3 x 5 lined cards; blank dividers, and celluloid tabs.[5] That will give you enough extra supplies so you can develop the system to cover some of your other needs.

In a minute I'll tell you how to use the cards. But first, you'll need to decide which household duties you can delegate to your children, assuming you still have teenagers or young adults in your home. Perhaps your husband can be included in the delegation of responsibilities.

Since we still have three children at home, Tom and I have divided the month into three sections and rotate duties every ten days. The schedule, which is kept on the inside kitchen-cupboard door, looks like this:

DATE	JOB & PERSON		
1st thru 10th	#1 Bath	#2 House	#3 Kitchen
11th thru 20th	#2 Bath	#3 House	#1 Kitchen
21st thru 31st	#3 Bath	#1 House	#2 Kitchen

#1—MIKE	#2—DEBBIE	#3—SHANNON

Once this schedule is set up, each child knows what his or her duty is and when it must be done. That way, they can plan

ahead for their own activities as well as the household responsibilities.

The 3 x 5 card file coordinates with this chart. Write each
day of the week on a separate tab and glue it onto the divider.
Three different-colored cards will go behind that divider, in-
structing child number one, two, or three exactly what needs to
be done on a specific day.

For instance, pink card: kitchen duties (list duties)
              blue card: bathroom duties (list duties)
        yellow card: house duties (list duties)

This is how it works: Each day, for example, whoever has
kitchen duty checks the card file when he or she gets home
from school. If outside activities interfere, the duty must be assigned to a sister or brother ahead of time; an IOU is put into
the box until it is made up.[6]

We don't have female and male roles in our home; we believe everyone needs to know how to run a household. This is
good preparation for their future, when they leave the nest and
must manage their own homes.

The card file and the schedule help eliminate the hassles that
usually develop when kids are asked to help out. With this
system there aren't any questions left unanswered. Only one
word of caution: If your family has not been in the habit of
sharing these responsibilities, let me suggest that you call
a family meeting and discuss the new plan. Then the kids can
offer their suggestions and feel part of the decision-making
process.

The second way we use the 3 x 5s in our kitchen is for menu
planning. Set up a section titled "Menus," with tabs for each
day of the week, as you did before. I have a rather flexible
menu planned for each day of the week so that the girls (who
are assigned cooking two nights each a week) don't have to
search for ideas. (Eventually our son will also cook. He turns
out a mean omelet now, usually a weekend treat.) This is how
the menu cards look:

MONDAY:	Leftovers and or hamburger casseroles, green salad.
TUESDAY:	Chicken—dumplings, oven-fried, sweet-sour, and so forth; vegetable, potatoes or rice, salad.
WEDNESDAY:	Crockpot (Begin before going to school) beef, chicken, chili beans, vegetable, potatoes, salad.
THURSDAY:	Cook's choice if not everyone is at home. Otherwise, fish—baked, broiled or roasted; potatoes, vegetable, green salad.
FRIDAY:	Spaghetti, lasagna, manicotti, tacos, enchiladas, and so forth; green salad.
SATURDAY:	Hamburgers, hot dogs or ?
SUNDAY:	Feast day: roast or ham and the works.[7]

This makes it simple for whoever happens to be cooking dinner that night. It takes a bit of planning. You must have all the food in your freezer or pantry.

These are only a couple of the ways the 3 x 5 card system can turn your household into an efficiently run organization. Another way to save time and be organized in the kitchen is with the use of a preprinted master grocery list. Make a list of all the foods you use. Either alphabetize them or arrange by your supermarket's aisle placement. Then have a number of these printed. When you run out of an item, all you have to do is check it off. At the end of the week, or whenever you shop, your list is already made up and waiting for you.

List making is something we have referred to many times throughout this book. It can be your best friend if you learn to use it regularly as a tool for achieving goals. I use a daily list the first thing in the morning so I know what I must achieve each day. I check things off as I go. If any items are left undone at the end of the day, they go on the top of the next day's list. I'd really be lost without this method of organizing myself.

To get yourself started toward developing this excellent habit, right now, list the things you must accomplish today:

1.   6.
2.   7.
3.   8.
4.   9.
5.   10.

Another way I organize and save time is by "packaging errands." I try to set aside a half day a week for running errands. My list comes in especially handy on that day, otherwise I'm liable to forget some of the things I wanted to accomplish. I may run to the market, stop by the cleaners, library, or printers, mail a package, and meet a friend for lunch. Packaging errands also saves expensive gasoline.

Even time in the car can serve double duty. I keep books there in the event I have to wait or get stuck on the freeway. I also keep a small notebook in my handbag as well as one in the car, so I can jot down thoughts as they come. Sometimes I can even write a short note to my daughter in Alaska, in what would otherwise be wasted time.

There are many ways to make time serve double duty, and you will develop these as you become more aware of time management and good organization.

One of the important things you'll want to include in your time-management program is a specific time each day for yourself. It's your growing time—a time to be alone with your thoughts, reading the Bible and other books of inspiration. It is a time for meditation. Perhaps you aren't familiar with that word, or it may frighten you. To me, meditation means to think quietly about what I've read, while God meets me in my subconscious mind and puts meaning to the words. There's nothing mysterious in it.

It is a time to nourish my soul—to replenish what I have used.

I believe it is vital for every woman to set aside a time—if only a few minutes each day—so she can communicate with God. I also find that praying the last thing in the evening and the first thing upon waking is a source of spiritual nourishment.

Spiritual nourishment, organization of time and activities, plus goal setting will help you develop your ageless attitude at forty-plus so that you can feel more fabulous today and always.

Assignment: **Charting Your Course**

1. Make a conscious effort to eliminate wasted time.
2. Plan constructive use of any newly found time.
3. Think about and set daily, short-term, and long-range goals.
4. Read *Sidetracked Home Executives* by Pam Young and Peggy Jones. Study their ideas for organization and adapt them to organizing your home. Set a goal of one month to get it accomplished.

Anyone who stops learning is old, whether this happens at twenty or eighty. Anyone who keeps on learning not only remains young but also becomes constantly more valuable.

HARRY ULLMAN

17

Sandra: A Feeling-Fabulous Success Story

I would feed you with the finest of the wheat, and with honey from the rock I would satisfy you.[1]

Before we talk more about using all the principles of goal setting and organization, I want to again impress upon you that your life is controlled by your thoughts. And your thoughts determine your goals. Because of this, you'll want to "let your thoughts develop a nostalgia for the future, instead of the past if you want to remain productive and vital. Develop enthusiasm for life, create a need for more life and you will receive more life."[2]

Developing enthusiasm for life and finding a life goal is not always the easiest thing to do at forty-plus. Many people have difficulty with it at any age. But at forty-plus, it becomes a crucial matter if life is to be fabulous in the future.

I have many friends and acquaintances whom I see struggling because they don't know what to do with their lives as middle age approaches. Right now, they aren't feeling fabulous for a number of reasons.

At forty-plus some face the prospect of going to work after raising a family, but have no marketable skills. Some are widowed, some divorced.

More than half of all married women are now working outside their homes. That leaves the other half facing the empty-nest problem immediately or in the near future. Many women have let that problem slip by without facing their feelings and substituting positive action.

I know substituting positive action can be difficult, especially if you've been a homemaker all your life and feel like a second-class citizen because of the nature of your work. I hope you don't feel that, but rather that your job has been appointed by God, who sees it as vital and holy.

But right now, the question for many women who are forty-plus is "What am I going to do with the rest of my life? I have thirty or forty years ahead and I don't want to waste them."

That was the question a good friend came to ask me some time ago. She was in a mid-life dilemma. Sandra was married, had a son in college, and twin daughters soon to graduate from high school. She had been working part-time as salesclerk in a large department store and knew she didn't want to clerk for the rest of her life.

Even though two daughters were still at home, Sandra was well aware of the letdown so many mothers experience after their youngest child leaves home. To prevent this, she wisely looked ahead, planning for her future.

One of the options Sandra saw was going back to college. She had two years of junior college before her marriage to Jack. When she thought about college, she was afraid. Like so many other women in mid-life, she thought she didn't have what it takes to be a student.

I was really excited about Sandra's going to college. She knew I would be enthusiastic, because I, too, had been a forty-plus college student for four years before I became a writer.

But Sandra was one step ahead of me. She *knew* why she was going to college (to become a nurse), whereas I had been there looking for a career because a goal was not yet in sight. I had experienced all the stumbling blocks Sandra feared—not knowing how to study, feeling alien on a campus traditionally occupied by "kids," and adjusting to a new role of college student while being a wife, mother, and homemaker. By the end of the first quarter, all those fears had vanished and were replaced by enthusiasm. I loved college.

Because of my experience, I could identify with Sandra's reluctance; but I encouraged her to meet this mid-life challenge. Some of the obstacles Sandra had to overcome were related to feelings of self-worth tied into the image of motherhood. With motherhood duty about to run its course, Sandra felt her net worth was also running out.

Sandra went through periods of depression when she worried about the kids leaving, not knowing what to do with her life, not having an adequate education, and seeing herself as worthless and homely.

When Sandra finished telling me how empty life seemed, I asked her if she'd be willing to try out the principles I've outlined in this book.

She said, "Yes! I'll try anything. I don't like where I am. I don't like myself right now, and I've got to do something. Where do we start?"

These are the steps we outlined for Sandra, and you can apply the same principles to your life as we go, according to your particular problem. You might want to jot down notes along the margins, mark the passages with a yellow felt pen, or make notes on a blank sheet of paper. You will get the most out of this exercise if you outline your life as I describe the attitude changes and goal setting for Sandra.

Step One

The inner you (recognizing the negative attitudes). Sandra was already aware of her negative attitudes about herself, so we didn't have to dig around for them. We listed those on a sheet of paper so she could see what she needed to work on as her first project of change. They were:

Destructive self-image (felt worthless)
No confidence in herself outside homemaking role
No short-term goals
No long-term goals
Saw herself as an unattractive, matronly woman

It's clear to see that Sandra was suffering from a severe case of middle-age doldrums. The anticipated empty nest was punching the panic button. "What will I do when the kids are all gone? How will I prove my self-worth then? Will Jack and I have anything to talk about? What would happen to me if Jack died or divorced me?" *Half* of those concerns are enough to cause depression, if not hysteria.

But Sandra was wise. She knew she must change her attitudes and her life if she was to be a vital forty-plus who feels fabulous. Right then, however, Sandra didn't feel fabulous at all.

Sandra and I talked about developing an ageless attitude and forming a solid self-image. She had a very willing spirit, so I knew she wouldn't have too much trouble changing, although the negative habits were going to hang in there as long as possible. After all, they, too, were forty-plus!

Once we recognized the attitudes that needed changing, we moved on to Step Two.

Step Two

Moving forward (getting rid of negative attitudes). One of the first things I did was share with Sandra how large a part God had played, and continues to play, in my life. I told her about how the Bible has so many positive affirmations that are good for a woman who is forty-plus and helps to shed negative attitudes. I also told her how prayer helps give me strength to make needed changes.

Sandra was already aware of so many of her negative attitudes that she had the first part of the battle won. It's when negatives have to be pulled into awareness that it takes more time to change. Sandra could see that the negative patterns would have to be broken. She would have to get strict control over her mind.

After explaining the flush method (see chapter two) to Sandra, she decided to flush her negatives down the drain every morning and night and as many times in between as possible. She'd replace those negative thoughts with positive, affirming statements of faith in herself and God.

I suggested she build a storehouse of positive attitudes by reading Norman Vincent Peale's *The Amazing Results of Positive Thinking*, *The Power of Positive Thinking*, or *You Can If You Think You Can*. In addition, I also recommended Cecil Osborne's books *The Art of Understanding Yourself* and *The Art of Becoming a Whole Person*.

Sandra also said she would diligently study each chapter of this book and apply the principles daily. She promised to read the Bible and practice believing that God really loves her just as she is—that she is a worthy person, capable and worthy of receiving all of God's gifts.

In order to accomplish this, Sandra set aside a half hour a day when she could be quiet and alone and meditate on inspirational insights for her life.

She promised to release her feelings of fear, failure, worry about her future, and negative self-image, and instead think with an ageless attitude.

Step Three

Making the transition (putting it all into action). As I said, Sandra was a willing participant. Many women do have willing spirits when they can see a deep need to change their lives in some way. If she hadn't, I'd have suggested she pray for a willing spirit and act as if she already had one (see chapter three).

In order to facilitate a better self-image, Sandra made a list of her positive qualities on one sheet of paper. On another she listed her negative ones, as I've suggested earlier.

After that was accomplished, Sandra was prepared to add to the negative list as more destructive attitudes surfaced. She also happily knew that her positive list would grow larger as she conquered each of the negatives. Sandra looked at this project as a positive challenge.

It's fun to watch a woman of forty-plus make excellent progress, but Sandra was so eager to surge ahead that she kept urging me to move on. I kept reminding her to work on one thing at a time. I was afraid she would become discouraged if she tackled too many changes at once. But she was impatient.

Because of her eagerness, we started the 21-day plan for change. After talking about her future, she decided she definitely wanted to go to college to prepare for a career. But she was scared. I suggested she work on the fear of going to college and the inferiority she felt about becoming a student.

For 21 days, every morning and every evening and every spare minute she had, Sandra worked consciously to change her attitudes from fear to faith and confidence. She talked to herself daily for 21 days. Her goal was to build positive attitudes so she would enter college with confidence. She would also be accomplishing her first goal: a major attitude change.

I kept reminding Sandra that it had taken forty years to develop her negative attitudes and not to become so impatient with herself. I urged her to love herself, as well as be patient and kind.

At the end of 21 days, Sandra had established a pattern of

believing she could be a successful student. She was able to recognize the fears as soon as they reared their ugly heads. She quickly bombarded those fears with faith in God and herself by repeating some of the positive Bible verses she had memorized. Working to wipe out the fear of going to college also erased the feeling of inferiority about becoming a student. As I explained to Sandra, it's seldom that we work on one isolated problem without wiping out several others.

One of the ways Sandra reminded herself to be positive each day was through the use of the 3 x 5 card system we discussed in the last chapter. She wrote several meaningful verses on each card and had a different card for each day of the week. If she was at home all day, she'd refer to them in the kitchen. When she went to work, she'd put the card in her pocket or handbag so she'd have ready ammunition in case the negatives attacked.

It's important to remember how deeply the negative patterns are engraved in our minds. Even though we may think we have the problem conquered, we mustn't be too surprised if it appears again.

That's what happened to Sandra. One day she called in tears. "I just can't go to college (sob, sob); I can't sign up in the fall; I'm scared. I'll just keep working at the store . . ." She thought she was ready to give up. But I knew Sandra better than that, and I encouraged her to trudge on. She finally understood what I meant when I said, "Use the act-as-if method and pretend a lot."

That was when she got a grip on herself and pushed ahead. We were both determined that Sandra's ageless attitude would become a permanent part of her. I reminded her it's only natural to falter along the way—that's the human side of us.

Just before her daughters' graduation, Sandra enrolled in college for the fall quarter. She gritted her teeth and "acted as if" she had always been a college student, with the confidence of a super-*A* quiz kid. (Inside she was shaking.)

Sandra had jumped an enormous hurdle. Short-term goal number one had been accomplished.

Before Sandra enrolled in college, I encouraged her to talk to the counselor in charge of "returning" women. There she was helped to find her line of interest and to keep her schedule light enough to handle comfortably; there were still home responsibilities to think about.

In the fall Sandra quit her job as a clerk and started classes. She had developed many solid patterns of positive thinking and established the beginning of her ageless attitude.

Sandra saw a glimpse of what I'd been talking about—that being forty-plus is a good time to feel fabulous, as long as your life has meaning and direction.

A new life was just beginning for Sandra, as it can for you.

Assignment: **How to Get the Most out of This Book**

1. On the following page is an outline to be used in developing your own ageless attitude and setting goals for your life. Cut it out or copy it on another sheet of paper. Use it as an outline as you apply the principles of this book to your own life.

   This outline is like a blank check. If you continue to leave it blank, it will be worthless to you. If you apply it to your life, it will become priceless.

Guide to an Ageless Attitude

Goal: *To be Forty-Plus and Feeling Fabulous by developing an ageless attitude that allows you to think positive and live a life based on your vitality, not your age.*

Step 1–The inner you: recognizing negative attitudes and listing them

Step 2–Moving forward: getting rid of negative attitudes
  Use flush method.
  Read positive books, the Bible.
  Learn to believe in yourself and God.
  List how you will accomplish this.
  List your positive verses; memorize your favorites.

Step 3–Making the transition: putting it into action
  Make two lists: positive qualities and negative qualities.
  Concentrate on replacing negatives.
  Reinforce positives.
  Use 21-day plan.
  List your program for change and your goals.

Lists to make:
  Daily activities
  One-day goals
  Short-term goals
  Long-term goals

Goals to accomplish:
  Exercise and grooming
  Time management
  Organization of household
  Delegation of household responsibilities
  Menu planning
  Packaging errands

Immediate goal to be accomplished and time allotted:

Consider the postage stamp ... its usefulness consists in its ability to stick to one thing until it gets there.

ANONYMOUS

18

Making It All Work for You

Hope deferred makes the heart sick, but a desire fulfilled is a tree of life.[1]

Changing lifelong habits of thinking and creating a new life-style requires a lot of conscious effort, as you just saw in the last chapter. That was only the beginning for Sandra. There was still much work to be done.

It was at this point in Sandra's life that goal setting was to take on vital meaning. She had been drifting along before. After all (she thought) you don't need a set of goals to be a mother and homemaker. They just kind of develop by themselves and push you into all sorts of daily activities. Who had time for short-term and long-term goals? Not Sandra.

That was past tense! Sandra had just made her first commitment to a long-term goal: college. In two years she would become a licensed practical nurse, and then long-term goal number one would be accomplished.

With that commitment, Sandra knew she was going to need several short-term goals. We sat down and talked about goals.

238

Sandra admitted her thought process had not included goal setting. But now, with her increased responsibilities, it was going to be vital. She also had to think about time management.

"Time management?" Sandra looked rather blank at this point. But I said, "Well, Sandra, if you're going to college full time, be a loving wife and mother and an efficient homemaker, you'll have to manage your time wisely." She sighed and nodded, but question marks filled her eyes.

I gave Sandra a copy of the time-management form in chapter sixteen and asked her to fill it out. Even though her time schedule would change in the fall, filling in how she had been using her time would give her a clue to wasted-time patterns.

She charted her time for seven days and then brought it back to me. We saw some real problem patterns that could thwart her new responsibilities and goals. She was a slow starter in the mornings and wasted half a day watching TV, sipping coffee, phoning friends, and then trying to decide what to do with the rest of the day.

Once Sandra saw the wasted hours, she decided to use my daily list-making system for organizing her day. With a list, she'd be able to see exactly what she must accomplish each day. She would write down each activity, then check it off when done. Those left undone at the end of the day would be written at the top of the list the next day and get top priority.

Getting organized was exciting to Sandra, although she shuddered at the thought of doing so many things before lunch. She had convinced herself she was a night person and thereby justified slouching around all morning in her bathrobe and slippers with her hair uncombed.

That behavior brought up another attitude change to make. It's almost impossible to have an ageless attitude and feel fabulous if you have to look at yourself and see Gravel Gertie staring back at you in the mirror.

Sandra just threw up her hands! But I could see by the twinkle in her pretty blue eyes that she was getting rather excited about seeing a whole new self-image emerging. I explained how I exercised, showered, dressed, combed my hair, and applied makeup before I ever leave my bathroom in the morning—and what a difference it makes in my attitude about myself. I suggested she also try it.

"Too many things to change," she'd moan. But like a trooper, she stalked ahead. It was exciting to watch an ageless attitude being born.

I gave Sandra a couple of weeks to get used to the idea of not wasting her mornings. Then we talked about the management of household responsibilities. I suggested she read *Sidetracked Home Executives* by Pam Young and Peggy Jones and use as many of their ideas as possible to organize her home.

I also suggested that Sandra make out a household-duty schedule similar to the one in chapter sixteen that we use in our home. That way, she would know what she had to do—and when; her daughters would also know how to plan their time. Summer would be a good time to get everyone used to the new routines before Sandra and the twins started junior college in the fall.

Installing the menu idea was Sandra's next move toward efficient organization in her home (see chapter sixteen). She asked the girls each to cook two dinners a week. That left only three for Sandra to cook. With the menus planned ahead of time, cooking became an easier task. All she had to do then was insure that the pantry and freezer were well stocked. Jack volunteered for that job.

Sandra could see that time management could solve many of the problems she had faced in trying to run her household. By the time Sandra packed up her books and walked through those college doors, she not only felt more sure about herself, her household was more organized than it had ever been. "I'm not running around in circles anymore," Sandra confided.

Packaging errands was the next thing our forty-plus college

student learned. On her least busy school day, Sandra ran all the errands she had accumulated during the week. With a list in hand, she'd run by the cleaners, pick up groceries, mail packages, buy gifts, or whatever needed to be done, before going home.

Of course, Sandra didn't want to lose contact with close friends even though she was making new ones in college, so she sandwiched in a lunch hour with a friend on the same day she packaged errands.

Sandra worked very hard to organize her life so that college would not be a heavy burden for herself or her family. One of the things that lightened her load was finding that being forty-plus was not a hindrance on campus. Her fears about feeling like an alien vanished. She found that one out of three students was a returning homemaker like herself, seeking an education. They, too, had experienced the fear of returning to school and feeling inferior because of their age.

It doesn't take long to see that, most of the time, fear is all in our head—a negative attitude that makes us believe we're scared.

Sandra found that through redirecting her thoughts and working at developing an ageless attitude, she had more energy to do many things she wanted and enjoyed, like spending quality time with her husband. It wasn't unusual to see Jack in the kitchen helping Sandra prepare dinner, chatting about all the events of their busy lives.

Sandra's life is a happy, success story—the kind we all enjoy hearing. But if she hadn't become aware of the destructive attitudes that were accumulating at forty-plus, she might have developed many ways to cop out on life; she might even be one of the 4 million alcoholic women who feel worthless and blunder aimlessly through life.

You have just been through the steps that changed Sandra from a disorganized, discontented woman without goals into one who has organized her time and home. She has set some short-term and long-term goals and is developing an ageless attitude so she can feel fabulous at forty-plus.*

You, too, can become another Sandra. You may want to go to college as she did, but it isn't absolutely necessary. You can apply these principles to anything you wish to accomplish with your life. Seriously consider the next twenty, thirty, or forty years when you set your long-range goals.

Goals are set by women at all stages of forty-plus. You may be perfectly content to remain a homemaker, but you still need to set goals and meet them.

One of the goals of many women is to become beautiful. But by forty-plus, most have given up. Some feel homely and because of it feel inferior to other women. These negative feelings also affect their goals, as well as their outer image.

As I said earlier, Sandra had felt her appearance was ugly, even though she has a gentle face with lovely blue eyes with long lashes. So far, she hasn't discovered the beauty of wearing makeup and fashionable clothing, but I am confident that will come as her inner beauty grows and she learns to like herself more.

I have waited to mention beauty until these final pages because I want to emphasize that real, *ageless beauty must first come from deep within.* It is an attitude about yourself that is reflected through every layer of skin and tells the world who you are. *It's your ageless attitude.*

That's not to say we need nothing more. To the contrary, I do everything I can to make myself more acceptable and nicer to look at. I want to reflect what I feel deep inside—that I am an accepted, loved, child of God. The makeup I wear, my hairstyle, the clothing I choose all create an image that is my ageless-attitude signature.

---

* You'll note that Sandra phoned me a lot during those crucial months. It's not because she was weak and needed someone to lean on, but rather that she did not have my total outline for change; I was still in the process of writing this book!

Through the years I have received many compliments about my appearance, which I try to receive graciously. I take no credit for my physical features; they were God-given.

At fifty-plus, I feel more alive and attractive than I ever have in my life. But as a child I felt homely and inferior to almost everyone. My short blonde hair was cropped in the traditional bowl cut. My clothes were from a mail-order catalog. In high school someone casually mentioned that I had a nice figure, and I couldn't believe they were talking about me. I did not feel I had any positive qualities then.

Those feelings carried over into my young-adult life. And I am thankful for them because they probably caused me to search for a deeper meaning to life.

I tell you this because I want you to know that I am no different from most other women. We all struggle to be beautiful. Some try to accomplish it with makeup, others look for an ageless attitude.

Some try both. In her book *The Image of Loveliness,* Joanne Wallace talks about her feelings of ugliness. She enrolled in a self-improvement course, lost weight, used makeup, and practiced better posture. She went on to become a professional model. But still something was missing from her life.

Joanne says:

> I began to realize that the inside of my head and heart were ugly. How could I be attractive to others when I was so aware of the ugliness in my soul? How could I be motivated to love others, as Jesus asked me to do, when I concentrated on their faults?
>
> Where was the sparkle in my eyes, the lilt to my walk, the genuine reaching out to others that would make me truly lovely?
>
> It was not to be found in makeup, posture, and clothing. I had concentrated on exterior beauty so much, and reserved no time for developing the inner me.[2]

And Joanne found, as I have, that you must ". . . be transformed by the renewal of your mind, that you may prove what is the will of God, what is good and acceptable and perfect."[3]

Yes, *a renewed mind is the key to an ageless attitude* at any age.

It's yours if you want it. Seize it. Once you have it, clutch it and never let it go.

Develop those positive attitudes that make you lovely and acceptable to yourself. When you like you, so will others. Then your ageless attitude, through the outer you, will proudly reflect that you are:

FORTY-PLUS AND FEELING FABULOUS.

For information about a Forty-Plus and Feeling Fabulous newsletter, seminars, workshops, or speaking en-
gagements by the author, write to:

Ruby MacDonald
P.O. Box 2997
Vancouver, Washington 98668

Source Notes

Chapter 1

1. Matthew 5:14, 16 (RSV).
2. Dieter Hessel, *Maggie Kuhn on Aging* (Philadelphia: Westminster Press, 1977), p. 13.
3. Thomas A. Harris, M.D., *I'm OK—You're OK* (New York: Harper & Row Publishers, Inc., 1973), adapted from chapter 2, pp. 39–59.
4. Gloria Heidi, *Winning the Age Game* (Garden City, N.Y.: Doubleday & Company, Inc., 1976), p. 8.

Chapter 2

1. Mark 9:23 (RSV).
2. *Webster's Seventh New Collegiate Dictionary* (Springfield, Mass.: G. & C. Merriam Co., 1961, 1966), pp. 57, 529.
3. Matthew 9:29 (RSV).
4. Philippians 4:13.
5. Matthew 9:17.
6. Matthew 11:28, 29.
7. 1 John 4:18.
8. Job 3:25 (RSV).
9. Norman Vincent Peale, *The Power of Positive Thinking* (Englewood Cliffs, N.J.: Prentice-Hall, Inc., 1956), pp. 124, 125.
10. Peale, *The Power of Positive Thinking,* pp. 124, 125.
11. Peale, *The Power of Positive Thinking,* adapted from chapter 9.
12. Peale, *The Power of Positive Thinking,* adapted from chapter 9.
13. Matthew 9:29; 17:20 (RSV).
14. Philippians 4:13 (RSV).

Chapter 3

1. 1 Corinthians 13:4 (RSV).
2. 1 Corinthians 13:4 (RSV).
3. Matthew 22:39.
4. Psalms 139:23 (RSV).
5. James 2:16 (RSV).
6. Psalms 139:13, 14 (TLB).
7. Cecil G. Osborne, *The Art of Understanding Yourself* (Grand Rapids, Mich.: Zondervan Publishing House, 1967), p. 153.
8. Osborne, *The Art of Understanding Yourself,* pp. 153, 154.
9. Maxwell Maltz, M.D., *Psycho-Cybernetics* (Englewood Cliffs, N.J.: Prentice-Hall, Inc., 1960), p. xv.
10. Maltz, *Psycho-Cybernetics,* p. 92.
11. Maltz, *Psycho-Cybernetics,* p. 28.
12. Maltz, *Psycho-Cybernetics,* p. 40.
13. Romans 8:31 (RSV).
14. Philippians 4:13 (RSV).
15. Luke 17:21 (RSV).

Chapter 4

1. Proverbs 17:22 (RSV).
2. John 8:32 (RSV).
3. Paula Weideger, *Menstruation and Menopause* (New York: Alfred A. Knopf, Inc., 1975), p. 196.
4. Louisa Rose, ed., *The Menopause Book* (New York: Hawthorn Books, Inc., 1977), adapted from chapters 1 and 2.
5. Gloria Heidi, *Winning the Age Game* (Garden City, N.Y.: Doubleday & Company, Inc., 1976), adapted from p. 224.
6. Weideger, *Menstruation and Menopause,* adapted from chapter 2, pp. 17–19.
7. Gloria Heidi, *Winning the Age Game,* p. 231.
8. Morris Fishbein, M.D., *Modern Home Medical Adviser* (Garden City, N.Y.: Doubleday & Co., Inc., 1956), p. 49.
9. Ecclesiastes 8:1 (TLB).

Chapter 5

1. Proverbs 8:11 (RSV).
2. *Information for the Patient,* Pamphlet No. 328 (New York: Ayerst Laboratories, Inc., 1980).

3. *Cancer Facts and Figures* (New York: American Cancer Society, 1981), p. 15.
4. *Cancer Facts and Figures,* p. 15.
5. Lila Nachtigall, *The Lila Nachtigall Report* (New York: G. P. Putnam's Sons, 1977), pp. 119, 120.
6. Nachtigall, *The Lila Nachtigall Report,* pp. 119, 120.
7. Nachtigall, *The Lila Nachtigall Report,* adapted from chapter 16.
8. Matt Clark and Mariana Gosnel, "Managing the Menopause," *Newsweek* (February 9, 1981), p. 92.

Chapter 6

1. 1 Corinthians 3:16 (RSV).
2. Hyman Jampol, *The Weekend Athlete's Way to a Pain Free Monday* (Los Angeles: J. P. Tarcher, Inc., 1978), p. 5.
3. Lila Nachtigall, *The Lila Nachtigall Report* (New York: G. P. Putnam's Sons, 1977), p. 157.
4. Jampol, *The Weekend Athlete's Way to a Pain Free Monday,* p. 30.
5. Jampol, *The Weekend Athlete's Way to a Pain Free Monday,* p. 34.
6. Jampol, *The Weekend Athlete's Way to a Pain Free Monday,* p. 35.
7. *Royal Canadian Air Force Exercise Plans for Physical Fitness* (New York: Simon & Schuster, Inc., 1974), pp. 16–18.

Chapter 7

1. Proverbs 31:22 (RSV).
2. 1 Peter 3:5.
3. Charles R. Swindoll, *Insight for Living* (tapes).
4. Swindoll, *Insight for Living* (tapes).
5. Carole Jackson, *Color Me Beautiful* (New York: Ballantine Books, 1981), p. 58.
6. Jackson, *Color Me Beautiful,* p. 58.
7. Joanne Wallace, *The Image of Loveliness* (Old Tappan, N.J.: Fleming H. Revell Company, 1978), p. 122.

Chapter 8

1. Proverbs 13:12 (rsv).

Chapter 9

1. Matthew 10:30, 31 (rsv).
2. Gloria Heidi, *Winning the Age Game* (Garden City, N.Y.: Doubleday & Co., 1976), p. 62.
3. Joanne Wallace, *The Image of Loveliness* (Old Tappan, N.J.: Fleming H. Revell Company, 1978), p. 84.

Chapter 10

1. Genesis 2:18 (rsv).
2. Matthew 7:24–27.
3. *Webster's Seventh New Collegiate Dictionary* (Springfield, Mass.: G. & C. Merriam Co., 1961, 1966), p. 167.
4. Ephesians 5:22–23 (rsv).
5. John Powell, *The Secret of Staying in Love* (Allen, Texas: Argus Communications, 1974), p. 127.
6. Powell, *The Secret of Staying in Love,* p. 128.
7. John Powell, *Why Am I Afraid to Tell You Who I Am?* (Allen, Texas: Argus Communications, 1969), adapted from pp. 54–61.
8. Powell, *The Secret of Staying in Love,* pp. 186, 187.
9. Powell, *The Secret of Staying in Love,* pp. 186, 187.
10. Cecil G. Osborne, *The Art of Understanding Your Mate* (Grand Rapids, Mich.: Zondervan Publishing House, 1970), p. 28.
11. Ecclesiastes 2:26 (rsv).
12. Osborne, *The Art of Understanding Your Mate,* p. 116.

Chapter 11

1. Proverbs 31:10 (rsv).
2. John Powell, *Why Am I Afraid to Tell You Who I Am?* (Allen, Texas: Argus Communications, 1969), adapted from pp. 65–79.
3. Acts 7:33 (rsv).

Chapter 12

1. Song of Solomon 7:10–12 (RSV).
2. Louisa Rose, ed., *The Menopause Book* (New York: Hawthorn Books, Inc., 1977), p. 112.
3. Ed Wheat, M.D., and Gaye Wheat, *Intended for Pleasure* (Old Tappan, N.J.: Fleming H. Revell Company, 1977), p. 104.
4. Wheat, *Intended for Pleasure,* p. 104.
5. David Reuben, M.D., *Everything You Always Wanted to Know About Sex But Were Afraid to Ask* (New York: Bantam Books, Inc., 1969), p. 49.
6. *Webster's Seventh New Collegiate Dictionary* (Springfield, Mass.: G. & C. Merriam Co., 1961, 1966), p. 172.
7. Wheat, *Intended for Pleasure,* p. 126.
8. Jason Towner, *Jason Loves Jane (But They Got a Divorce)* (Nashville, Tenn.: Impact Books, 1978), p. 150.
9. Genesis 1:31.
10. Charles R. Swindoll, *Strike the Original Match* (Portland, Ore.: Multnomah Press, 1980), p. 73.

Chapter 13

1. Matthew 6:14 (RSV).
2. Paula Weideger, *Menstruation and Menopause* (New York: Alfred A. Knopf, Inc., 1976), pp. 196, 197.
3. Weideger, *Menstruation and Menopause,* pp. 196, 197.
4. Louisa Rose, ed., *The Menopause Book* (New York: Hawthorn Books, Inc., 1977), pp. 130, 131.
5. Rose, *The Menopause Book,* pp. 130, 131.
6. Matthew 19:6 (RSV).
7. Jim Smoke, *Growing Through Divorce* (Eugene, Ore.: Harvest House Publishers, 1976), p. 25.
8. Smoke, *Growing Through Divorce,* p. 25.
9. Cynthia Scott, "Does Your Church Treat Divorced People Like Criminals?" *Moody Monthly* (September 1981), pp. 10, 11.
10. Scott, "Does Your Church Treat Divorced People Like Criminals?" pp. 10, 11.
11. John 4:7–26.
12. Jeremiah 30:17 (RSV).

13. James Allen, *As a Man Thinketh* (Old Tappan, N.J.: Fleming H. Revell Company, 1980).
14. Ephesians 5:23 (RSV).
15. Psalms 30:5 (RSV).

Chapter 14

1. Matthew 6:15 (RSV).
2. Mel Krantzler, *Creative Divorce* (New York: New American Library, 1975), p. 70.
3. Krantzler, *Creative Divorce,* p. 71.
4. Krantzler, *Creative Divorce,* adapted from pp. 94, 95.
5. Harold Ivan Smith, *A Part of Me Is Missing* (Eugene, Ore.: Harvest House Publishers, 1979), p. 45.
6. Smith, *A Part of Me Is Missing,* p. 45.
7. Morton Hunt and Bernice Hunt, *The Divorce Experience* (New York: McGraw-Hill Book Company, 1977), p. 140.

Chapter 15

1. Psalms 23:6 (RSV).

Chapter 16

1. Jeremiah 29:11 (RSV).
2. Alan Lakein, *How to Get Control of Your Time and Your Life* (New York: New American Library, 1973), p. 37.
3. Lakein, *How to Get Control of Your Time and Your Life,* p. 31.
4. Peggy Jones and Pam Young, "No Longer Locked Out, Left Behind or Overdrawn," *The Columbian* (June 22, 1981).
5. Peggy Jones and Pam Young, *Sidetracked Home Executives* (New York: Warner Books, Inc., 1981), adapted from p. 38.
6. Jones and Young, *Sidetracked Home Executives,* adapted from chapter 4.
7. Jones and Young, *Sidetracked Home Executives,* adapted from p. 147.

Chapter 17

1. Psalms 81:16 (RSV).
2. Maxwell Maltz, M.D., *Psycho-Cybernetics* (Englewood Cliffs, N.J.: Prentice-Hall, Inc., 1960), p. 240.

Chapter 18

1. Proverbs 13:12 (RSV).
2. Joanne Wallace, *The Image of Loveliness* (Old Tappan, N.J.: Fleming H. Revell Company, 1978), pp. 153, 154.
3. Romans 12:2 (RSV).

Suggested Reading

Part I

Allen, James. *As a Man Thinketh.* Old Tappan, N.J.: Fleming H. Revell Co., 1981.

Harris, Thomas A., M.D. *I'm OK—You're OK.* New York: Harper & Row Pubs., Inc., 1969.

Heidi, Gloria. *Winning the Age Game.* Garden City, N.Y.: Doubleday and Co., Inc., 1976.

Maltz, Maxwell, M.D. *Psycho-Cybernetics.* Englewood Cliffs, N.J.: Prentice-Hall, Inc., 1960.

Kanin, Garson. *It Takes a Long Time to Become Young.* New York: Berkley Publishing Corp., 1979.

Osborne, Cecil G. *The Art of Becoming a Whole Person.* Waco, Tex.: Word, Inc., 1978.

Osborne, Cecil G. *The Art of Learning to Love Yourself.* Grand Rapids: Zondervan Publishing House, 1976.

Osborne, Cecil G. *The Art of Understanding Yourself.* Grand Rapids: Zondervan Publishing House, 1968.

Parker, William R. *Prayer Can Change Your Life.* Englewood Cliffs, N.J.: Prentice-Hall, Inc., 1957.

Peale, Norman Vincent. *The Power of Positive Thinking.* Englewood Cliffs, N.J.: Prentice-Hall, Inc., 1954.

Part II

Heidi, Gloria. *Winning the Age Game.* Garden City, N.Y.: Doubleday and Co., Inc., 1976.

Kaufman, Sherwin A. *The Ageless Woman.* Englewood Cliffs, N.J.: Prentice-Hall, Inc., 1967.

Nachtigall, Lila. *The Lila Nachtigall Report.* New York: G. P. Putnam's Sons, 1977.

Weideger, Paula. *Menstruation and Menopause.* New York: Alfred A. Knopf, Inc., 1975.

Part III

Cooper, Mildred, and Cooper, Kenneth H. *Aerobics for Women.* New York: M. Evans Co., Inc., 1972.

Heidi, Gloria. *Winning the Age Game.* Garden City, N.Y.: Doubleday and Co., Inc., 1976.

Jampol, Hyman. *The Weekend Athlete's Way to a Pain Free Monday.* Los Angeles: J. P. Tarcher, Inc., 1978.

Royal Canadian Air Force Exercise Plans for Physical Fitness. New York: Pocket Books, Inc., 1974.

Wallace, Joanne. *The Image of Loveliness.* Old Tappan, N.J.: Fleming H. Revell Co., 1978.

Part IV

McGinniss, Alan Loy. *The Friendship Factor.* Minneapolis: Augsburg Publishing House, 1979.

Morgan, Marabel. *Total Joy.* Old Tappan, N.J.: Fleming H. Revell Co., 1977.

Osborne, Cecil G. *The Art of Understanding Your Mate.* Grand Rapids: Zondervan Publishing House, 1970.

Powell, John. *The Secret of Staying in Love.* Allen, Tex.: Argus Communications, 1974.

Powell, John. *Why Am I Afraid to Tell You Who I Am?* Allen, Tex.: Argus Communications, 1969.

Shedd, Charlie, and Shedd, Martha. *Celebration in the Bedroom.* Waco, Tex.: Word, Inc., 1979.

Swindoll, Charles R. *Strike the Original Match.* Portland, Ore.: Multnomah Press, 1980.

Wheat, Ed., M.D., and Wheat, Gaye. *Intended for Pleasure.* Old Tappan, N.J.: Fleming H. Revell Company, 1981.

Wright, H. Norman. *Communication: Key to Your Marriage.* Ventura, Calif.: Regal Books, 1979.

Part V

Krantzler, Mel. *Creative Divorce.* New York: New American Library, 1975.

Smith, Harold Ivan. *A Part of Me Is Missing.* Eugene, Ore.: Harvest House Pubs., Inc., 1979.

Smoke, Jim. *Growing Through Divorce.* Eugene, Ore.: Harvest House Pubs., Inc., 1979.

Smoke, Jim. *Suddenly Single.* Old Tappan, N.J.: Fleming H. Revell Co., 1982.

Towner, Jason. *Jason Loves Jane (But They Got a Divorce).* Nashville: Impact Books, 1978.

Part VI

Bliss, Edwin C. *Getting Things Done.* New York: Charles Scribner's Sons, 1976.

Bolles, Richard Nelson. *What Color Is Your Parachute?* Berkeley, Calif.: Ten Speed Press, 1981.

Hensley, Dennis E. *Staying Ahead of Time.* Indiana: Research and Review Service of America, 1981.

Lakein, Alan. *How to Get Control of Your Time and Your Life.* New York: New American Library, 1974.

Lenz, Marjorie, and Shaevitz, Marjorie Hansen. *So You Want to Go Back to School.* New York: McGraw-Hill Book Co., 1977.

Loeser, Herta. *Women, Work and Volunteering.* Boston: Beacon Press, 1974.

Winston, Stephanie. *Getting Organized.* New York: Warner Books, Inc., 1980.

Young, Pam, and Jones, Peggy. *Sidetracked Home Executives.* New York: Warner Books, Inc., 1981.